The Economic Era of Health Care

The Economic Era of Health Care

A Revolution in Organized Delivery Systems

Everett A. Johnson

Montague Brown

Richard L. Johnson

Jossey-Bass Publishers • San Francisco

Substantial discounts on bulk quantities of Jossey-Bass books are available to corporations, professional associations, and other organizations. For details and discount information, contact the special sales department at Jossey-Bass Inc., Publishers (415) 433–1740; Fax (800) 605–2665.

For sales outside the United States, please contact your local Simon & Schuster International office.

Manufactured in the United States of America on Lyons Falls Pathfinder Tradebook. This paper is acid-free and 100 percent totally chlorine-free.

Library of Congress Cataloging-in-Publication Data

Johnson, Everett A.
  The economic era of health care : a revolution in organized
delivery systems / Everett A. Johnson, Montague Brown, Richard L.
Johnson.
      p.   cm.—(The Jossey-Bass health series)
  Includes bibliographical references and index.
  ISBN 0–7879–0284–5 (alk. paper)
  1. Integrated delivery of health care—United States. 2. Managed
care plans (Medical care)—United States. 3. Hospital trustees—
United States. I. Brown, Montague. II. Johnson, Richard L.
(Richard Lee), date. III. Title. IV. Series.
RA410.53.J64 1996
362.1'0973—dc20   96–14448
                                                           CIP

HB Printing 10 9 8 7 6 5 4 3 2 1   FIRST EDITION

Contents

Preface

The Economic Era of Health Care is the end product of numerous conversations among and articles written by its three authors. Our concern in testing our thoughts and ideas with each other centered on developing an understanding of what is happening in health care. As we identified issues, we shared our ideas by exchanging papers that we prepared as a way of clarifying and interacting with each other. The results of these discussions and exchanges of ideas have been categorized to make up the chapters of this book. Our intention is to communicate with our colleagues about the developments now underway in health care. The author or authors of each chapter are identified for the reader's information.

Three strands of health care activities that traditionally developed independently are now converging in the emerging era of concern about the costs of medical care. Hospitals developed out of religious and charitable functions to care for the poor and the ill, independent of physician activities. The family doctor of the turn of the century has become today's primary care physician, specialist, or hospital-based physician. Blue Cross, established in the 1930s, has led to the growth of large commercial insurance companies, health maintenance organizations (HMOs), preferred provider organizations (PPOs), and the government programs of Medicare, Medicaid, and CHAMPUS. These three functions—Blue Cross, commercial insurance companies, and government programs—represent success stories of health care, and collectively they have become so essential that the public is now insisting on greater accountability for their services.

These functions arrived at their current stages of development largely through independent routes and over different time frames. They are at a point where they are viewed by the public as requiring coordination, and a new trend of integrated organizations is perceived as necessary to achieve quality care at a reasonable cost. The goal of bringing the three separate functions together in a coordinated whole faces a challenging set of circumstances. Hospitals are technological institutions that are costly to operate and that require major capital investments on a routine basis. Medical practice has proliferated into numerous specialties composed of individual practices, single specialty groups, and large multispecialty clinics. Blue Cross and indemnity insurance carriers have become HMOs and other managed care plans with a wide variety of payment and coverage strategies that bewilder the public and confuse their decision making. Trying to put all three functions into a coordinated program in the competitive marketplace is akin to attempting to put Humpty Dumpty back together after he has fallen off the wall.

Providers of medical care services have reacted to this perceived need for coordination by combining into larger organizations. Independent practitioners are forming independent provider organizations or combining practices into one corporate entity, while for-profit companies are raising large equity funds to acquire physician practices, on the premise that for-profit companies are the key to managing health care costs. Hospitals are forming affiliations and buying other institutions in an attempt to force managed care plans to contract with hospitals as the hospitals improve productivity by creating economies of scale. Successful managed care plans are buying out competitors and purchasing hospitals and physician practices in order to gain greater control over their providers in the marketplace.

Because of the turmoil now occurring, the health field is reorganizing and regrouping into larger and larger corporate structures, with the predominate type of ownership remaining an open question. Traditionally, most hospitals have been not-for-profit corporations; the for-profit hospitals have accounted for approximately ten percent of all hospitals. Physician practices, by contrast, have always been for-profit. Prepaid health care programs, beginning with Blue Cross in the 1930s, have been not-for-profit because they have been sponsored by community not-for-profit hospitals. However, when for-profit commercial insurance companies entered the prepayment arena, they introduced experience rating, coinsurance, and deductibles in order to undercut the pricing structures of Blue Cross. To maintain market position, Blue Cross began to use experience rating and adopted the strategies of the commercial carriers. The commercial insurance companies eventually emulated the Kaiser system of managed care and capitation. The Blues responded by forming for-profit subsidiaries to handle nontraditional lines of business. Currently, the ten largest HMOs have a total of 20.9 million members: the for-profits have 13.6 million members, and the not-for-profits have 7.3 million, of which 6.6 million are enrolled in Kaiser Permanente.[1] These ten HMOs have accumulated reserves of $10.5 billion, of which not-for-profit HMOs have $1.681 billion, and for-profit HMOs have $8.856 billion or the equivalent of $651.18 per member.

The question of how these large reserve funds will be spent is important, and several options come to mind. Large HMOs may use the money to purchase smaller HMOs in their effort to expand their membership base, or the money may be used to acquire physician practices in order to further penetrate a market. Some HMOs may even buy hospitals in their market in order to increase control of the HMO's cost of operations. These efforts will be made to avoid pressure from employers and state insurance commissions to lower premium charges. To expand markets or better control the cost of providers, HMOs will prefer spending reserves to reducing premium rates.

Under these evolving conditions what strategies will hospital executives and their governing boards undertake as countermeasures? Will they continue as major players on the health care scene? Will nonprofit hospitals be able to compete successfully against the deep pockets of managed care plans with huge reserves? Will practicing physicians be able to maintain their independence, even if merged into large multispecialty groups? Will doing good ultimately triumph over doing well financially? Who will be the winners and who will be the losers a decade from now?

The future can be shaped and molded, but to do so requires understanding of present trends and where they might lead. If inadequate attention is devoted to understanding the likely outcomes of the course of events, the future is already cast in concrete. This book is about the future of health care, the problems to be solved, the threats that must be met, and the opportunities that lie ahead for those hospitals and physicians willing to challenge the status quo.

Realigning Roles

As the days unfold in the last decade of the twentieth century, the health field is experiencing traumatic times that are likely to continue well into the next century. The specter of capitation as a way of paying for health care is the driving force behind all of the changes now taking place, and has resulted in the development of two major trends. For the first time in the history of health care, the primary concern has shifted away from medical care considerations to economic considerations. Coupled with this has been the recognition by providers (physicians and hospitals) that "mom and pop" operations are no longer viable and that it is now necessary to aggregate the provider side of health care into larger and larger units in order to offset the economic strength of managed care plans.

When the concern shifted from medical care to economics, the basic foundation of health care was shaken to its roots. No longer were the providers in control of all the decisions about health care. Employers, business coalitions, government, and managed care plans began to exert increasing influence through payment mechanisms. What had been accepted as the prerogatives of providers came under fire from the payers, who no longer regarded health care as something from which they were excluded and whose role was limited to paying for whatever were determined to be the costs of care.

The expansionist era that had been underway for four decades drew to a close. Optimism about the future was replaced with fear, a growing concern that mere survival in the new era would be a challenge and that a number of hospitals in nearly every city would eventually be closed. No longer was there a widespread belief that next year would be better. As the number of persons enrolled in managed care grew, competition increased commensurately. The view of hospitals as friendly adversaries was replaced with a climate of hostility engendered by the increasing competition for market share. The concept that capitation puts providers at full risk developed out of the payers' desire to control their expenditures for health care.

As the economic era develops and matures, new concepts will be introduced and tried. Advocates will claim results before all the evidence is in as to whether they are effective or not. As the old problems disappear, they will be replaced with others that are new, different, probably of greater complexity, and associated with greater risk.

Up until the beginning of the economic era, risk taking was minimal. A hospital might lose, but never to the point of being forced out of business. Physicians were all winners—some bigger winners than others, but nevertheless, all winners. Today, the health care climate is increasingly risky, which poses great difficulties for those who have been risk-averse as a result of past conditions.

The instrument employed in bringing about the economic era is managed care, which is viewed by many payers as a way of controlling the costs of health care without interfering with the quality of care. Whether this is true or not remains to be seen. Because the economic era emerged only within the late 1980s, the full ramifications of its impact on the health field will not be known for at least a decade. Only in time and with experience will it be possible to evaluate the value of managed care in achieving the desired results.

Contents of the Book

The first part of this book is devoted to an examination of economics as more important than health care services. The chapters in this section review how the emerging primacy of economics will be regarded by a public that has long held as most important the quality of the medical care they receive. These chapters examine the role of managed care and the massive infusion of investor capital in buying hospitals, managed care organizations, and physician practices in the drive toward regional and national restructuring of insurance, hospitals, and physician practices. Included is a chapter on the economic credentialing of physicians—evaluating how effectively they use resources, as part and parcel of evaluating their overall effectiveness—and how such credentialing is likely to play out in a setting in which physicians have long been accustomed to being credentialed only with respect to their clinical skills. Finally, this section considers the ethical dimension of the economic era.

Part Two of the book takes a hard look at the development of managed care in the United States. This section responds to the widespread interest in capitation by asking whether it is a long-term solution to the cost of health care or a passing phenomenon that has such significant limitations that it will eventually be replaced by something else. The question of what might follow is also examined. In an attempt to understand how providers survive in a capitated environment, a chapter is devoted to considering alternatives. Also contained in this section is a description of how the public may ultimately come to view capitation, and an assessment of the role of managed care in community wellness and prevention as part of developing the responsibilities of managed care.

In a managed care scenario, the role of the physician is markedly altered. The distinction between primary care physicians and specialists is widening as a result of the types of payments made to physicians. The outcome is expected to be a substantial shift of physicians into primary care, resulting in an increase in the number of primary care physicians and a decrease in the number of specialists. The chapters in Part Two address the anticipated extent of these changes in physician manpower, and they look at how physicians and hospitals are organizing themselves to deal more effectively with managed care plans. In this new environment, a whole new set of tensions are developing that heretofore have not been encountered by many providers. The development of PHOs has led to an examination of the long-term viability of this type of organizational arrangement. A chapter is devoted to assessing the viability of PHOs as, like other new developments occurring in the health field, a long-term answer to the organizational needs of providers. Finally, although it is not in the forefront of current concerns, the impact of managed care on ethical considerations is a topic whose time will be coming; it is therefore anticipated in the last chapter of this section.

Since the beginning of the twentieth century, hospitals have become the dominant player in the health care arena, with 40 percent of all health care expenditures being spent by hospitals. In the emerging economic era, this balance will change as health care moves away from the freestanding community nonprofit hospital and shifts to organized delivery systems and managed care. The community general hospital will no longer be center stage, nor will it have the degree of influence it once had. Adjusting to its new role will require a reexamination of traditional values and roles that have evolved in the governance of institutions. How governance is affected is the theme of Part Three of this book. The chapters in this section explore the challenge to hospitals' abilities to remain not-for-profit corporations in light of the need for growth of the corporation and the aligning of physician interests with those of the hospital.

Part Four begins by considering the question of retreading hospital chief executives into system leaders. Chapter Sixteen discusses how the metamorphosis can take place that enables busy executives deeply enmeshed in their roles to make the transition from a hospital setting to a more broad-based health care organization. The chapter considers the requirements for success, as well as the reasons that there may be significant fallout among present-day hospital chief executives.

The next chapter presents an analysis of the skills required by physicians who become executives in the corporate setting, whether in managed care operations, hospital management, or health care system management, or in the new type of organization that may combine the three major components—hospitals, physicians, and managed care—in one corporation. The development of physicians as executives is a topic of interest because of the necessity of weaving together clinical and managerial skills. Clearly, there will be opportunities for physicians at both senior executive and chief executive levels in health care systems. The career path from clinical training and practice into the executive suite is a subject whose time has arrived, so it is discussed in this section.

Health professionals all proclaim an interest in the promotion of health, and while much is done by those in the healing professions and by hospital and managed care executives to promote health, the bulk of resources are devoted to cure rather than to prevention—to disease rather than to health. Managed care financing may even reduce the little bit of financial resources going into community health. This issue is also explored in Part Three.

Finally, Part Four examines four perspectives of key professionals. Traditionally, graduate education for health care management focused on the skills required for becoming the chief executive of a freestanding hospital. It was assumed that a graduate would initially be exposed to the world of hospitals through an administrative residency, followed by entrance into the general administrative ranks at a junior executive level. This would lead to positions of increasing responsibility and authority until, some two decades later, the ultimate position of chief executive would be obtained. With the development of organized delivery systems and the growth of managed care plans, however, the traditional curriculum for health care leaders is no longer relevant and has to be broadened to encompass new knowledge.

Conclusion

Much of what lies ahead in health care is unexplored territory. The ways of the past are being discarded so rapidly that what has proven to be of value may be lost. It certainly seems to be true that what led to the development of the American health care system as the finest in the world has many values and attributes that need to be retained. What should be kept and what should be discarded is the subject of the authors' concerns. All has not been well in the American health system, but neither has it been so out of touch with reality that the existing system should be tossed aside without giving due consideration to what has served the American public well. At the same time, the health care professionals who have made the system what it is must be willing to respond to the world as it is and not cling to a past that is no longer viable. Finding the pathway that saves what is useful and discards the concepts and attitudes that no longer apply is the test that is now under way.

Acknowledgments

For the past year, the three authors of this book have been actively engaged in a serious discussion and exchange of papers about the future of health care in this country. The results of our efforts became this book. In the course of this undertaking, we tried out our thoughts on a number of others, to whom we are indebted for their thoughtful responses and comments. Primary among these persons were our frequent collaborators, Jewel Johnson, Barbara McCool, and Sandra Gill. Additional feedback was received from

Robert Toomey, Pat Groner, Dennis Barry, William Bates, and Thomas Weil, as well as the editors of *Health Care Management Review.*

Note

1. Anders, G. "Money Machines: HMOs Pile up Billions in Cash as Analysts Wonder What They Will Do with It." *The Wall Street Journal,* December 21, 1994, p. 1.

June 1996

Everett A. Johnson
Atlanta, Georgia

Montague Brown
Tucson, Arizona

Richard L. Johnson
Chicago, Illinois

About the Authors

Montague Brown is editor of *Health Care Management Review,* chairman of Strategic Management Services, Inc. (SMS), and a consultant on strategy. He devotes his time to speaking on industry trends and governance organizational issues, and writing articles and books at his desert base camp near Tucson, Arizona. His current work is devoted primarily to a new book dealing with the widespread corporatization and commercialization of health care. This writing builds on insights gained from thirty years of active teaching and consulting on issues of strategy, vision, vertical integration, and governance.

Brown holds an A.B. degree and an M.B.A. degree from the University of Chicago, and a Doctor of Public Health degree and a Juris Doctorate from the University of North Carolina. He has held full-time research and teaching positions at the University of Chicago, Northwestern University, and Duke University, and adjunct positions at the Universities of Kansas and Oklahoma. Brown frequently lectures to students at a variety of universities.

Everett A. Johnson has been director of the Institute of Health Administration at Georgia State University since 1979. His career began in 1951 when, after receiving a B.S. degree from Northwestern University and an M.B.A. degree in hospital administration from the University of Chicago, he became administrator of Chicago Memorial Hospital. In 1954 he became administrator of the Methodist Hospital of Gary, Indiana. During his twenty-two years in Gary, the hospital expanded from 209 to 470 beds and added a second hospital of 165 beds in Merrillville, Indiana. From 1952 to 1976 he maintained a relationship as preceptor and lecturer with the graduate program in health care administration at the University of Chicago, from which he received a Ph.D. in 1962.

From 1977 to 1979 he served as associate director of the graduate program.

During his career, Johnson has been a committee and council member of the American Hospital Association and has served in its House of Delegates and on its nominating committee. He is a life fellow in the American College of Healthcare Executives, for which he has served as regent, governor, and chairman. He has been a member of the board of directors and executive committee of Blue Cross/Blue Shield of Indiana and of Georgia. He was the founding president and a member of the board of directors of the National Council of Community Hospitals. In 1968 he received the Tri-State Award of Merit, and in 1968 and 1973, the Edgar C. Hayhow Award for the Article of the Year. In 1989 he received the Silver Medal Award of the American College of Healthcare Executives. He has published more that eighty articles and four books.

Richard L. Johnson is former chairman of the board and cofounder of TriBrook Group, Inc. During his health care career he has served as assistant superintendent of the University of Chicago Hospitals, and as associate director of the Graduate Program in Hospital Administration and assistant professor of the Graduate School of Business at the University of Chicago. He was director of the teaching hospitals and associate professor in the School of Medicine at the University of Missouri. Johnson served as an assistant director of the American Hospital Association (AHA). Upon leaving the AHA, he joined the management consulting firm A.T. Kearney & Company, where he was vice president in charge of health field activities and a member of the board of directors. In 1972, Johnson and two of his colleagues formed the management consulting firm of TriBrook Group, Inc., in Oakbrook, Illinois. He served as president of the firm from 1972 through 1994, and then for two years as chairman. He has published more than 150 articles and five books.

Johnson has been a life member of the American Hospital Association; a fellow of the American College of Health Care Executives; and a fellow of the American Association of Healthcare Consultants and past chairman of the group. He has been awarded the Silver Medal by the American College of Hospital Administrators, and has received the Award of Merit from his colleagues in the American Association of Healthcare Consultants. He served as health advisor to the Secretary of the U.S. Air Force from 1986 through 1988, and he is a founding member of the Certified Management Consultants. He holds an MBA degree in Hospital Administration from the University of Chicago and a B.S. in zoology from Northwestern University.

The Economic Era of Health Care

Part One

Introduction

Chapter One

The Economic Era of Health Care

Richard L. Johnson

The roots of the current deep public interest in reforming the nation's health care system reach back to the turn of the twentieth century. Over the course of decades, care for the sick and dying has moved from inpatient care in a hospital setting to a loosely coordinated system of inpatient and outpatient ambulatory and hospital services. Health care services are valued activities that are now regarded as so important that they are seen as necessities that must be available to all individuals. The unquestioned desirability of having immediate access to health care stands as a testament to both physicians and hospitals. The nonavailability of health care services is no longer acceptable to the public.

An avalanche of health care proposals has been unleashed on the public, not only at the federal level but by state governments as well. In addition, purchasers of health care have formed coalitions at the local level, companies have become self-funded for health care, and third-party carriers have developed new and innovative financial arrangements for contracting for health care. Clearly, a new era in health care is under way that has evolved from and builds on the shoulders of the two previous eras of the twentieth century: the charitable era and the technological era.

The *charitable era* began at the turn of the century. It lasted for approximately fifty years, ending shortly after World War II. During that period, hospitals became recognized by the public as institutions that could provide care to alleviate some illnesses and that were needed as a community resource. At the same time, various religious groups recognized that owning and operating hospitals was in keeping with the ministry of healing, and even hospitals that were nonreligious recognized a community responsibility to provide care and were organized as nonprofit entities.

People believed that a hospital had a responsibility to care for all who needed hospitalization. The theme of charitable services dominated the development of nonprofit hospitals. The economic depression of the 1930s reinforced the need for hospitals to provide charity care, and fund-raising drives by hospitals emphasized the role of charity. If deficits occurred, board members were expected to make up the difference.

The *technological era* of health care began following World War II, when advances in medical technology began to be felt in hospitals. The opportunity to specialize in clinical fields led an increasing number of medical school graduates to seek additional training in residency programs, which accelerated the transformation of the nonprofit hospital from a charitable institution into a technological enterprise. Accompanying these clinical developments was the rapid introduction of management systems into hospitals as the result of graduate-level education in health care organization and management. As more and more professional health care executives joined the ranks of hospital management, financial operations were tightened and budgets were put in place. Governing boards no longer relied on donations and fund-raising drives. At the same time, the amount of charity provided became more tightly controlled as management was faced with larger and larger capital expenditures in order to keep up with the growing sophistication of technology. By the end of the 1980s, the transformation had taken place—hospitals had become technological enterprises, still nonprofit, but organizationally behaving as any large corporate entity.

As the technological era evolved, charity care was replaced substantially with two federal programs, Medicare and Medicaid, designed to pay for hospital care on behalf of the elderly and the poor and needy. Because these two programs do not now pay hospitals the full cost of the care they provide, hospitals subsidize these patients by charging higher-than-cost to patients who are either self-pay or covered by commercial insurance. In a very real sense, charity care in hospitals has been replaced with cost shifting. Knowing their costs and revenues in a detailed manner, hospitals have been able to keep up with the required capital expenditures through larger and larger bottom lines.

By the time 1990 rolled around, the technological era was winding down. Hospitals had become technological enterprises that funded capital expansion through the debt market. Public fund-raising drives were no longer a significant source of capital. Capital needs and balanced budgets had become the driving forces. Management was responding with larger and larger bottom lines and larger and larger cash reserves that made the bond market comfortable in making loans for ever increasing amounts to nonprofit hospitals.

Telltale signs of things to come had begun to develop in the 1980s, when 10 percent of the acute beds were owned and operated by for-profit health care companies. By 1990, these companies were not only using debt for expansion, but they were also relying heavily on equity markets. In addition, managed care was becoming well-known to the public as more and more employers turned away from commercial insurance and traditional Blue Cross plans. As this trend continued, physicians began forming *independent practice associations* (IPAs) and *preferred provider organizations* (PPOs) that would offer discounted rates to large-bloc purchasers of health care. As the hue and cry from corporations, individuals, and government grew louder about the ever increasing cost of health care premiums, organized efforts developed among payers concerned with limiting the annual price rises they were experiencing.

The Dawn of the Economic Era

By 1990, the economic era had developed enough steam that it could be characterized by consolidation and competition. This era is now in its early stages. Its hallmark will be economic enterprises built on the foundation of medical care that developed out of charitable concerns. The day of the freestanding hospital and the solo practitioner is being replaced with systems of hospitals and group practices of physicians as they aggregate their services. The "mom and pop" era of health care is rapidly drawing to a close. As might be expected at this stage of development, a variety of approaches are being taken that will likely end up with the same outcome. The resulting organization that can be anticipated fifteen to twenty years from now is the for-profit *organized delivery system* (ODS). Each ODS will be composed of hospitals, primary care physicians, and specialists, and will be financed by a prepayment plan. Physicians will play a central role in the ODS, and because physicians' practices are for-profit, the ODS will adopt this form of corporate organization. While such a system will be focused at a local level, it may have an overarching prepayment arm that encompasses a number of local ODSs as part of the same corporation. Since for many communities the large multibillion-dollar health care corporation lies years in the future, the intervening years will be filled with an array of differing organizational attempts by health care organizations to become larger and more encompassing.

The driving force in health care in the emerging era is competition, brought about by the underlying economics, not by inadequacies in the ability to provide satisfactory medical diagnoses and treatment. In this new era, while those providing health care services have a desire to retain existing profit margins, those paying for health care have for the moment taken the initiative because of their major interest in limiting expenditures. Business corporations have concluded that the best method for limiting premium expenditures is to offer health care providers large blocs of care for bidding on a competitive basis. As a result of corporate interests, corporations have a preference for signing health care contracts with prepayment organizations, which offer managed care options utilizing primary care physicians as gatekeepers, who must see patients first before authorizing them to see a specialist. This approach reduces the use of hospital and physician services. Having determined that the use of a gatekeeper has economic advantages to the buyer, corporate purchasers have recently begun to express interest in having providers bid for contracts that combine both professional services and hospital care in one price for an episode of illness. This interest is now leading payers to push for a monthly payment per subscriber, or *capitation*. By thus "capitating" providers, the economic risk is borne by those providing health care service, and the payer's own economic exposure is limited. The desired end result is for the payer to be able to control all elements of the payment for health care service. For this to be successful, hospitals and physicians must ultimately become *closed-staff* organizations, which limit the number of positions in specialty and clinical departments.

Bypassed in the race to develop widespread capitation plans has been the concept of connecting the episode of illness with some degree of patient economic responsibility for the care that is received. Providers are being made financially responsible for the services provided to patients while, as long as the monthly subscriber rate is paid, the patients have no responsibility. The theory behind this approach is that it will force providers to reduce costs because they are at economic risk. Also implied is that the quality of care and its availability will at least remain at existing levels. Whether this occurs or not is an open question.

Developing a series of events that will culminate in a closed system is unlikely in most communities. Such events will take place in major cities, where giant prepayment organizations will do battle with each other for market share. Hospitals and physician groups will be pawns in a high-stakes prepayment game. Even if in the next few years hospitals link with groups of physicians to form large multispecialty groups, these groups will be no economic match for prepayment organizations controlling hundreds of millions of premium dollars annually. In smaller cities the pattern is likely to be less structured and never to reach the stage found in major metropolitan centers. Nevertheless, as physicians recognize that managed care is on their doorstep, events can be expected to transpire rapidly in even small towns and cities, but varying organizational relationships will emerge. Competition among managed care plans is apt to be missing in small towns and cities because of insufficient volume, leaving the playing field open to competing physician groups or competing hospitals.

Managed Competition and Collaboration

At present, the health care buzz words in popular usage are "managed competition" and "collaboration." The belief among those paying for health care services is that managed competition offers the best solution for effectively blunting annual premium increases in health care coverage. Recognizing the overwhelming interest in this subject, health care providers are busily developing collaborative arrangements so as to be able to offer "seamless" care when bidding on managed care contracts. The development of solid working relationships between hospitals and physicians is being defined as a collaborative process, one in which both parties recognize a mutual dependence. This movement into a physician-hospital organization (PHO) or ODS, which is a variation of the PHO, is one in which hospitals and physicians are joining together because they both see the need to do so for economic survival. Among many hospital and medical staffs, the arrangement is voluntary, in response to the marketplace. To date, sufficient thought has not been given to how to hold these parties together when bidding conditions become difficult and revenues scarce. In the rough and tumble of a competitive environment in which economic stakes become higher and higher, the need will quickly surface for binding contractual relationships between the parties to the PHO or ODS. Penalty clauses will become part and parcel of PHO and ODS organizations, in order to ensure that the PHO or ODS will continue to service the contracts obtained from prepayment organizations or self-insured corporations.

In the decades since World War II, the health field has not experienced widespread conditions in which there are winners and losers. Physicians and hospitals had long been accustomed to a risk-free environment in which there were only winners, some bigger than others, but no losers, which makes learning to live in a competitive environment a difficult lesson. In the unfolding health care environment, there is expected to be a surplus of both specialist physicians and hospital beds, leaving a considerable imbalance between supply and demand among these providers. This disparity will give purchasers a golden opportunity to exploit the imbalance for their own economic interests. A "shakeout" among providers can be anticipated, which will cause many internal tensions and disputes among the partners in PHOs and ODSs.

In a truly competitive environment, the purchaser will be unconcerned with the fallout to providers. As long as a sufficient number of hospitals and physicians survive to provide acceptable levels of service, the focus in health care will remain economic. As a result of this continuing focus, the alliances and affiliations (which are weak organizational structures to begin with) that lose the bidding wars will break apart as each member strives to develop its own marketing strategy in order to survive. Penalties for breaking away from an alliance or an affiliation will be insignificant compared to the potential loss of revenues and the consequences—such as the firing of personnel, inability to make loan payments, and so on—that result from the loss of a managed care contract.

Market Capacity

In a marketplace that has excess capacity, the aggregation of providers into large economic units is an important strategy because size increases clout. By itself, however, this approach is not enough. Within a provider's organizational structure, the ties binding the various parts together must be strong, in order to withstand the internal tensions that will inevitably arise as a result of there being far more suppliers of services in the marketplace than demand for services.

When a provider organization responding to a request for a proposal becomes aware that a successful bid must be below the organization's current cost of operations, physician providers will expect the hospital to take the necessary hit, and the hospital, likewise, will expect its partner, the physicians, to be the losers. Dealing successfully with this type of internal tension requires not only strong leadership but also having in place significant economic penalties. All of the provider participants must understand the price to be paid if they fail to accommodate to the realities of the marketplace.

While it is important at this stage of consolidated competition to form these collaborative provider organizations, the goodwill of the parties involved is insufficient. Goodwill merely opens the door to the formation of the PHO or ODS. Once a PHO enters the competitive marketplace, its leadership needs to have the authority to commit the organization, even in circumstances that may not be desirable. To continue to rely on the goodwill of participants as the only organizational mechanism for securing acceptance of necessary negotiating decisions in a tough marketplace will likely result in a breaking apart of the provider organization.

The widespread belief that managed competition offers the best route to meeting people's health care needs in a cost-efficient manner has led to a rush among providers who fear they may be left out when the new health care system falls into place. The providers—physicians and hospitals—are assuming that the marketplace will be the balancing mechanism for the available supply of physicians and hospital beds and the demand for the hospital's services. However, the effort to put together the various provider pieces will result in many variations based on economic perceptions. Quite often, physicians do not view the hospital as a partner of choice, preferring to deal only with physicians. When confronted with managed care, specialists quickly appreciate that primary care physicians control the flow of patients, and the specialists become anxious to ensure a continuation of referrals from their primary care sources. This may lead to attempts to form multispecialty groups, to lock primary care physicians and specialists into the same physician organizations. Combining a number of existing practices into one physician corporation requires considerable capital funds, which may be beyond the financial capabilities of many specialist organizers and which therefore may lead them reluctantly back to including the hospital in the corporation as well.

In some communities, primary care physicians may elect to form their own corporation and take capitation but exclude specialists from joining the group. Taking control of capitation puts primary care physicians in a position to dictate the terms under which they will use selected specialists. This might take the form of asking specialists to bid for contracts, and keeping the specialists at arm's length. In addition, a group of primary care physicians, or a combination of primary care and specialist physicians acting as a PPO, might elect to seek competitive bids from hospitals and then contract with the lowest bidder. To do so would put the PPO into the position of taking all of the risk, not just for physician services but for the hospital as well, a difficult position in the event that the hospital successfully refuses capitation and opts for a per diem or a per case method of payment.

At the present stage of development, the efforts of hospitals and physicians are being directed toward finding partners and developing arrangements that will enable providers to bid on managed care contracts with federally sponsored programs, state initiatives, local business coalitions, or existing carriers offering a managed care option. Putting together provider health care conglomerates is the immediate focus of attention and will continue for the next few years.

At the moment, there is much jockeying among providers for the best position. Specialists are trying to capture primary care physicians in order to protect their referral patterns, and primary care physicians are just recognizing their pivotal role and attempting to avoid being captured by other specialists and hospitals while at the same time maximizing their newfound economic value. Hospitals are seeking to use their economic strength to build systems that will enable them to grow and prosper. Underneath all of these efforts by providers is a recognition that fundamental changes are needed, and while there may be serious differences of opinion about how best to achieve the needed changes, this recognition is shared by the payers for health care services.

The Changes Needed

Providers and payers generally agree that the following elements are needed in the provision of health care services:

1. Guaranteed access for all persons
2. A minimum standard of benefits for everyone
3. A standard reporting form
4. Choice of physician and hospital, but perhaps limited by choice of plan
5. No denial of coverage for preexisting conditions
6. Protection of existing standards of quality of care and, to the extent possible, improvement of those standards
7. Rehooking of an episode of illness with a degree of economic consequences for the patient, but use of capitation as a method for achieving this result

The root of the problem in providing health care services is not in the quality of care but rather in the means of paying for and financing health care. The issue is economic—the provider wants to protect income, the payer wants to limit expenditures. Providers also have an additional set of problems as the result of the growth of managed care. Hospitals appreciate that managed care plans reduce the number of days patients spend in the hospital, which leads to a need for fewer inpatient beds, and ultimately to a reduction in the number of hospitals. Specialists, who account for 70 percent of all practicing physicians, are well aware that managed care uses substantially fewer specialists, and that as this approach to providing health care develops, there will be an overabundance of physicians in specialty fields. Conversely, primary care physicians recognize that they are increasingly in short supply and stand to gain economically under managed care. Providers thus have a legitimate concern about how economics may impact their ability to provide care.

Consequences of Ill-Founded Economics

A prevailing concept among the payers of health care is that annual increases in the costs of coverage have to be reined in. Unspoken is the belief that this can be accomplished without a lowering of quality of care or a decrease in access to medical care. The belief that quality and access are not affected by restricting payments to providers is akin to believing in the tooth fairy.

In bringing economics to the forefront in health care, both government and third-party payers are trying a variety of approaches to focusing their attention on restricting payments to providers. At the federal level, payments to hospitals have shifted over time from cost reimbursement to per diems to per case payments. The Clinton administration has proposed capitation with overall control of expenditures at the national level through caps on monthly premiums. At the same time, managed care plans are resorting to seeking competitive bids from hospitals and patients for large blocs of patients.

The concept of managed competition is gaining favor with increasing frequency. Seemingly unrecognized, however, is that when competition is managed, it is no longer competition. Managed competition implies controls or limits. The "unseen hand of the marketplace" is no longer unseen, but rather has a defined boundary. Where the boundary is set determines the economics that apply. If the boundary is set too low and a hospital cannot stay within the limit, market forces are disrupted, which is already a problem with the Medicare and Medicaid programs, which provide payments that are substantially below the operating costs of hospitals. Even though this is true, the Clinton administration has indicated that it wishes to further reduce projected spending levels in excess of $200 billion over the next few years for these two programs.

With rapid growth in managed care, the application of a boundary will drastically impact institutional decisions, which may not be in accord with public expectations. Payers should not assume that quality of care standards will remain at present levels, nor should they assume that hospitals and physicians will provide unrestricted access in the event that the established boundary is below operating cost levels. Up to now, hospitals have accepted Medicare and Medicaid below operating cost levels because they could shift costs to other payers. However, as the number of patients grows under managed care, hospitals will have increasingly fewer opportunities to use this method, and the time to make tough decisions will have arrived. Physicians likewise will be making equally tough decisions.

The Effects of Capitation

With capitation as the likely method of payment for primary care physicians, two behavior patterns may emerge. Since capitation pays a primary care physician a fixed monthly amount per subscriber whether or not a medical service is provided, a physician may be inclined to work only a set number of hours per day per week, since the amount of money received will be the same whether the physician works forty or sixty hours per week. With primary care physicians now in short supply, and the shortage projected to continue indefinitely, the end result will be longer and longer queue lines for patient appointments. Some primary care physicians will probably develop nine-to-five practice hours, except for true emergency patients. Under capitation, the physician enjoys no economic reward for working twelve or fourteen hours per day, or six or seven days per week.

The other behavior pattern occurs when the capitation payment to a primary care physician is less than what might be paid from another source, such as a self-pay or more liberal health insurance payment policy. The patients payed for by capitation will have longer waiting times. Patients covered by the more liberal payment plans will be given preference, and their waiting times will be less than those covered by capitation. If the physician employs a nurse practitioner, patients covered by capitation may have to be seen by the nurse practitioner before being seen by the physician, while those with preferred payment sources may not have to see the nurse practitioner first. Removing the economic incentive that is a built-in part of fee-for-service medical care takes away the motivation for working sixty or seventy hours per week. Since the mean number of hours worked per week by a family practitioner has been 58.5 hours, and for internal medicine practitioners, 62.2 hours per week,[1] a decision to reduce work hours to forty hours per week would require a one-third increase in the supply of primary care physicians in order to provide the same coverage to patients.

Capitation also has a downside for hospitals. In a competitive marketplace dominated by capitation, conventional wisdom is that putting hospitals at risk for their services benefits the public economically. This is true, but only to the extent that the economics of "going at risk" are stable over a period of several years. Where capitation has been successful and hospital utilization has fallen dramatically from one year to the next, the hospital is unlikely to retain the same capitation rate. It is safe to assume that for a hospital that is under contract with a managed care organization and that has provided fewer services or cared for fewer patients in a given year, the managed care plan will adjust the capitation rate downward at the end of the contract period.

The ideal model for capitation is usually envisioned as a managed care plan—hospital services, specialists, and primary care physicians all in one economic unit. However, when all of these components are contracted separately by the managed care plan, the economics are not the same. When each group has a separate contract with the managed care plan, the hospital is in no position to affect the use of its facilities, because the volume is controlled by the physicians, whose economic interests are not the same as the hospital's.

When capitation is the basis of payment to providers, the payer can ignore the volume of services provided, and their cost. The responsibility for determining volume of activities is divided among the various providers. Implicit in capitation is the assumption that enough dollars are being paid to the providers so that they can render adequate care if they judiciously use the health care resources. This is a more workable plan when the component parts—hospital, primary care physicians, specialists, and prepayment plans—are all in the same corporation. In an integrated entity, whatever is financially adverse for one of the components carries over to the corporation as a whole. When the linkages between the components are by contract, however, the economics are markedly different. For example, as long as a hospital can engage in cost shifting, the problem of inadequate payment can be ameliorated, but when the point is reached that average cost instead of marginal cost must be applied, hospitals have to face reality.

Risk Shifting

When a managed care plan contracts with hospitals, primary care physicians, and specialists, the risk is totally shifted away from the managed care plan and becomes the responsibility of the providers. The only risks to the managed care plan are complaints about provider services. If enough complaints are made by enrollees about how they are treated, the managed care plan may have to consider contracting with other providers at contract renewal time. If only the same restricted choices are open to the managed care plan, it may be forced to increase its capitation rates in order to reattract providers. However, when an offered capitated rate is below the average cost for providing service, providers can be expected to bid in anticipation of providing only minimum services. When the managed care plan offers contracts with stipulated outside maximum limits, the bidding providers will first ascertain whether the boundary permits a reasonable rate of return. If it does not, the bidders will treat the maximum limit as a minimum, and all bids received will be at the outside limit, if bids are received at all.

To the extent that providers may be paid for services with fees controlled by the federal government, experience with the Medicare and Medicaid programs indicates that the managed competition limits will be set by federally driven budgets and not by quality-of-care concerns. It is likely that federally set boundaries will also lead the way for nongovernmental payers. Under such circumstances, hospitals would be forced to take a number of steps that may include

- Drawing down cash reserves
- Deferring capital expenditures
- Using nonoperating revenues to meet operating expenses
- Reducing the number of personnel
- Reducing fringe benefits of employees
- Improving control of nonpersonnel operating expenses

These steps present both opportunities and difficulties. When hospitals can improve on efficiencies, the payment system will be used as the justification for doing so. However, difficulties will occur in those hospitals in which the intensity of illness has steadily risen over several years. Intensity factors primarily affect nursing services, so significant increases in intensity should be reflected in growth in the number of nursing hours per patient day, with a commensurate increase in nursing salary costs. However, when revenues have bumped against a ceiling and no further revenues are in sight, the only choice open is to hold the line on costs and let the quality of care slip.

Under capitation, the intensity-of-illness factor is likely to escalate at an even more rapid rate than it has over the past few years, due to the effort to keep patients out of the hands of specialists and hospitals. Inpatients are likely to be very ill when admitted, and require more services, not fewer. As the intensity of illness increases, nurses must spend more time at the patient's bedside observing physiological changes. If this does not happen, the patient's condition may deteriorate or the patient may die. Physicians' awareness of what can happen makes them worry about their patients—and about getting sued for malpractice.

Where the ties that bind primary care physicians, specialists, and hospitals to a managed care plan are separate capitation contracts, the ability to cope with risk is seriously flawed. At its heart, the use of capitation assumes that the volume of services provided can be standardized and controlled to predictable levels. A corollary assumption is that when managed care plans use economic penalties, any deviations beyond the established boundaries will result in corrections to bring unanticipated surges in volume back to established norms. The benchmarks typically being used are those of managed care plans that have used capitation for many years, such as Kaiser-Permanente. Plans that are attempting to achieve similar results need to remember that not only is Kaiser-Permanente a single economic unit but it also has a common culture of medical care that has evolved over decades. In the development stages of a PHO or ODS, no such culture exists. Physicians in solo practice, small single-specialty groups, or small multispecialty groups lack familiarity with budgeted volumes of activity and will expect the management of the hospital to deal with the financial aspects of overages. When all providers have separate contracts with the managed care plan, no one contractual party feels fiscal responsibility for the other contractual parties if they encounter economic problems with their capitated rates. The unaffected parties may be, and probably will be, sympathetic to the beleaguered partner and take what steps they believe are reasonable, but without seriously affecting their own financial status. In this type of situation, it is not the responsibility of the contractual partners to bail out the party that may be in financial trouble.

Conclusions

Now that the health care field has commenced its journey into the economic era, the question is whether or not concerns about cost and access will replace the long-standing goals of quality, comprehensiveness, and availability of medical care. If cost and access become paramount, will the present standards of care be maintained?

To date there appears to be a general belief that if all of the health care eggs are put into the capitation basket, the problem of escalating costs will be contained while maintaining adequate access and quality of care. This belief is fostered by the history of the evolution of health care during the last one hundred years, from the charitable era through the technological era to the present early stages of the economic era. This history is an unparalleled success story that is expected to continue. Physicians have been the driving force in this evolution because for decades they have consistently placed the obtaining of solid clinical results ahead of cost.

For generations physicians have been taught, and have practiced, to place the patient's well-being first and leave the financial aspects of care to be handled at the end of the episode of illness. Recognized or not, that premise is now under challenge. Capitation requires the physician to balance clinical judgments with economic realities. In effect, capitation states, "Doctor, do whatever you believe is clinically necessary, but understand that the costs incurred are not the responsibility of the patient or the managed care plan. They are your responsibility, because you have accepted a fixed amount of money each month in return for care, whenever needed and in whatever amount is required."

In the relationship between managed care plans and providers, the providers bear all of the risk and the prepayment organization is primarily a conduit for funds. Over time this will turn out to be an unsatisfactory relationship because the risk is one-sided. When this one-sided relationship becomes widely recognized by providers, they are likely to terminate their relationship with the managed care plan and form their own plan, or they may be bought by the managed care plan to form one economic unit. In either approach, the cost of forming the new organizational relationship will require a major commitment of capital dollars in order to align the components in a way that maximizes profits for those involved in ownership, as well as to create a more efficient system.

If it is necessary, in working out these arrangements, to raise equity money (which is likely), the leverage for influencing the decisions of the newly formed organization is most likely to shift from Main Street to Wall Street. When that shift takes place, the emphasis will move from a concern for community good to a concern for shareholder dividends. Large amounts of money will be involved, including both assets and revenue streams, that will make health care increasingly attractive to the financial world. Table 1.1 provides an example of what is taking place. Fifteen percent taken off the top of the premium revenue dollars ($420 million) for administrative costs, taxes, reserves, and profits will amount to $63 million per year. When for-profit organizations have a "spill-off" of that amount of money, it will attract equity investors. Results of this magnitude will be possible on an enrolled population base between 400,000 and 500,000 persons. On a population base of 250 million, the potential is five hundred times greater, or approximately $2.1 trillion of revenue and a 15 percent margin of $31.5 billion.

Table 1.1. Managed Care Plan X.

Number of Participants	Premium/Month	Premium/Year	Total Annual Premium
100,000 families	$300	$3,600	$360M
50,000 singles	$100	$1,200	60M
150,000			$420M

The conclusions are indeed obvious, because the magnitude of potential profits is going to attract a great deal of attention. Whichever organization controls the premium revenue dollars is going to control the provider resources, and if the controlling organization is for-profit and therefore has shareholders, community good will take a back seat to dividends. Such a thought is anathema to those who have devoted their careers and lifetime efforts to nonprofit hospitals. However, it is a possibility that must be realistically faced.

The tide of change is sweeping the health care field into uncharted waters. If providers find themselves excluded from the overarching decisions being made by either government or the financial world and do not take the initiative to control or substantially influence what takes place, the end result will be a disillusioned public. So far, the existing health care system has been shaped by the providers. Tomorrow, the health care system is most likely to be shaped by government and investors seeking dividends. Controlling costs and increasing access to health care may well be achieved, but the price for achieving these results will be paid by the public. They will have to deal with a provider system that has been forced to respond to a drummer not of its choosing. Instead of patients' needs coming first, the demands of government and investors will take over and patients will come to realize that the health care system as they knew it no longer exists.

Finally, the question of the inevitability of this outcome needs to be addressed, and whether alternatives might be possible must be considered. If providers continue to put their own specialized interests first and are willing to sacrifice their provider partners on the altar of their own economic gain, then the interests of the payers will prevail. But if providers are able to put aside their differences and develop meaningful relationships with users of health care services, they may find a way to protect the values that the public has come to appreciate. To be successful, primary care physicians, specialists, and hospitals need to put together meaningful organizations that engender employer and public support. This will be a tough task requiring determination, flexibility, and a strong awareness of the consequences of failure.

The odds are against providers laying aside all of their differences and developing meaningful dialogues with business coalitions, self-funded corporation plans, and other user groups. The odds favor those providers with large amounts of money and deep pockets that come from revenue streams of monthly premium payments by many subscribers in capitation plans. It is too early to determine the outcome. A decade from now we will know who won and who lost.

Note

1. American Medical Association. *Physician Marketplace Statistics, 1992.* Chicago, Ill: American Medical Association, 1992, p. 31, Table 2, "Hours In All Professional Activities Per Week, 1992."

Chapter Two

Mergers, Networking, and Vertical Integration

Montague Brown

Hospitals, physicians, insurers, and managed care firms are networking, merging, and forming horizontally and vertically integrated organizations to finance and deliver health care. Organizations, investors, health professionals, governments, and other groups such as alliances, hospitals, medical societies, group practices, and so on are positioning themselves to gain or preserve market share, income, revenue, and power in a radically agitated marketplace. Power and control in the health care enterprise are shifting, threatening to topple traditional institutions even as these institutions try to reinvent themselves into what their leaders think will be the most logical inheritor of power in the future. The word "power" is used here to mean control, authority, and the ability to make things happen. Physicians, hospitals, managed care firms, traditional insurers, and the individuals controlling such organizations are pursuing strategies that they each hope will position them to have substantial power. The fact that not all of them can occupy the same space simultaneously accounts for many of the attempts to establish networks and other loose forms of affiliation.

Note: This chapter has been adapted from Brown, M. "Mergers, Networking, and Vertical Integration: Fear and Fascination with Managed Care and Investor-Owned Hospitals Drive a Revolution." *Health Care Management Review,* 1996, *21,* 29–37. Copyright © 1996, Aspen Publishers, Inc. Used with permission.

Where is the health care field going and what does all of this shifting herald? We are seeing the elaboration of the next generation of organizations that hope to solve the riddle of providing affordable, accessible, quality health services for all Americans; or we are in the middle of a transition that holds additional surprises just up the road. What is driving the field toward integration and consolidation?

A central thesis of this chapter is that ideas have power. People who lead institutions are doing things that they think will position their organizations for success in a changed world of health care. Their ideas of what major changes are necessary to make health care more affordable are what motivate them to reposition their organizations. Much of the change of the past thirty years has been based in large part in expectations of how managed care will evolve and how provider institutions will compete. Ideas help to explain why people pursue networks and alliance building. For many voluntary hospitals, the ideas of networking, alliance building, mergers, and vertical integration are conditioned by expectations of what investor-owned institutions and aggressive managed care firms can and will do with their access to equity market capital. (Investor-owned institutions have done many things well over the years, but they have come only recently to regional integration. Now that they have moved in this direction, corporations such as Columbia/HCA are moving aggressively—going after tertiary referral hospitals to complement their networks in all regions where they aspire to have a major presence.)

Managed care and investor-owned institutions with access to new equity capital have been powerful motivators for many voluntary and governmental hospitals to find competitive strategies for coping. Ideas have ranged from loose affiliation to total consolidation under single ownership, and the most recent iteration of collaboration, the merging of physicians with hospitals. Ultimate ideas run to putting managed care, hospitals, and physicians under one corporate control. Naturally, each competitor envisions its group leading this new integrated entity. The struggle for power and control accounts for many of the failures to create successful alliances, networks, and mergers.

The argument that fear of managed care, investor-owned hospitals, and entities capitalized by market equity does not negate the fact that many hospital executives believe that vertically integrated regional organizations are desirable and likely to be more effective than the current fragmented model. What hospital executives argue is that without the threat of loss of power and control, they would not be able to convince their medical staffs and trustees that the risk and cost of building such systems would be worthwhile. Change involves trauma, so it is helpful to have a real threat of greater trauma if the present institution's "insiders" fail to change first. For many executives the task is to balance legitimate fears with ideas for desirable and workable kinds of organizations by building more efficient and affordable health care delivery systems.

This chapter approaches the subject of collaboration from the perspective of how managed care, competition with investor-owned hospitals, and other elements of health care delivery have impacted the trends noted so well in the many reviews of this subject presented elsewhere.[1]

Background

Any starting point for consideration of a subject as broad as networking and alliances is somewhat arbitrary. Hospital associations grew after World War I and got another big boost during the days of Hill-Burton facilities financing. Many of these associations built additional shared services. The rationale for the national alliances getting so much attention today is that they were built to give one group of hospitals a competitive advantage over their neighboring hospitals. Most hospital association efforts included all local hospitals and were called shared service programs. All of the hospitals involved could benefit from the association. Current alliances for the most part consider competitive advantage to be a major deciding factor in admitting members and designing programs.

When Medicare and Medicaid were enacted in the mid 1960s, the health care industry geared up for heady growth. For many Americans, this enactment heralded the promise of health care as a right, with government picking up the tab for the elderly and poor. New York and California each exceeded the Johnson administration's Medicaid cost estimates for the nation. The new plans, with their mandate to continue fee-for-service payment to physicians and cost-plus reimbursement for hospitals, seemed to forecast a steady increase in money and practically a federal guarantee for whatever it would take to make an investment in health services profitable.

As the promise of cost-plus reimbursement for hospitals and universal coverage came into play, entrepreneurial physicians and others were able to convince equity market players that the industry would be a gold mine for investor capital. Medicare led many hospitals to be rebuilt, making it attractive for physician-owned institutions to use equity funding. The investor-owned hospital chain flourished. Growth in the South, Southeast, and West, where for-profit hospitals already existed, soon became the regions with greatest for-profit chain growth. Many small hospitals that had been built with Hill-Burton federal funds sold out to the developing chains, which then scrapped obsolete plants and built modern hospitals. Many large, well-established not-for-profit hospitals found themselves competing with these firms. For-profit chains took over marginal hospitals, replaced them with first class facilities, and began recruiting physicians who had been key players in the not-for-profit hospitals.

By the early 1970s the need for cost containment was evident; the federal government had underestimated the costs of Medicare and Medicaid but was unwilling to pay hospitals their costs of operation, so providers were forced to find ways to contain costs. Shared services, especially group purchasing programs, became popular mechanisms for deflecting public criticism about cost increases in hospital budgets. By publicizing the savings realized from these programs, hospitals were letting the public know that they shared the public's concerns about cost. Health planning— by which hospitals had to seek approval from a state agency for expenditures over $1 million or risk not receiving Medicare payments—attempted to curtail duplication of costly technologies. New capital flooded the market and competition increased, but the solutions did not seem to be working. During this period, the idea arose of using health maintenance organizations (HMOs) to contain costs. This idea was based on an older concept of prepaid group practice. At first, adoption was slow, but many knowledgeable professionals agreed that it would take an approach with strong economic incentives for physicians to keep costs down and for patients to accept the discipline of such regimes. By the 1980s, both managed care and investor-owned hospitals had built in scale advantages by becoming involved in national purchasing programs and by using standardized methods for building and operating hospitals. (Chains did not benefit from the purported advantages of scale for purchasing until the mid 1980s. Many authors have noted that these chains benefited greatly from their ability, like all hospitals, to price their product to produce the profits required for their business. This is changing, but it provided a solid basis for growth throughout the 1970s and 1980s.)

In the 1970s, the nation tried price controls, voluntary efforts, and other slogans to contain health care costs. Shared purchasing grew from state hospital association efforts to national alliances built outside the political structure of hospital associations. A number of these national alliances merged—and indeed, the merger of these giant purchasing organizations continues today (for example, the merger between American Health Systems and Premier Alliances, which resulted in $500 million annual purchases from Johnson & Johnson (J&J), making the combined organization J&J's biggest customer.[2] Look out little niche companies, when elephants dance they can be dangerous.) A comprehensive assessment of alliances is presented by Zuckerman, Kaluzny, and Ricketts.[3]

The promise in hospital mergers and consolidations was that if the number of owners were reduced, then hospitals could plan more rationally and reduce the duplication of high-cost technologies in individual markets. Shortell and others studied many of the systems built out of mergers and concluded that many of the promises of such systems have not been realized.[4] The potential exists, but it has not been fulfilled.

Many reasons for this failure have been asserted and speculated upon. Getting a larger share in adjacent markets locks in sufficient scale to justify more complex procedures that require access to large population bases. If the market has strong competitors, there is pressure for price and cost reduction. Many systems, however, have gained major advantages from mergers and consolidations without having to go through the more difficult task of rationing programs and services among their owned hospitals.

Before antitrust laws were applied, hospitals planned voluntarily, with each hospital sorting out what it would do and what others would do. This behavior was encouraged by health planning agencies that evolved out of a long history of voluntary planning in which collaboration and sharing aptly described typical hospital behavior. As long as each hospital got the programs it wanted, voluntary collaboration worked well. Even when every hospital did not get everything it wanted, there was usually an explicit or implicit quid pro quo for the "losing" organizations. (I would not, of course, argue that everyone was satisfied with voluntary dividing up of markets. Those who have gotten the heart programs in such divisions have done very well, much to the chagrin of those who have gotten behavioral units.)

Dividing markets through agreement became a verboten topic once antitrust laws were applied directly to the health care field.[5] When agreements to fix price or divide markets[6] became illegal, it became necessary to look at total integration as a means to achieve collective, regional action. Multihospital systems were spawned during the 1970s,[7] after the antitrust moves dampened the ability of hospitals to voluntarily assign markets and roles; then, local and regional mergers increased.

The growth of managed care during the 1980s accelerated in the 1990s, becoming the force behind physician alliances, hospital mergers, and national and regional hospital alliances. Providers were driven by the thought that managed care firms would eventually narrow their provider lists to those that were most efficient in the delivery of a comprehensive range of services. It is theoretically possible for managed care firms to sign up only the best providers and leave others off their preferred-provider lists. That the reality might not have caught up with the theory did little to stop attempts by providers to form their own networks. From the beginning of the formation of the large voluntary hospital alliances, competitive advantage in competing local networks was a prime factor. (While studying one of the early multihospital systems in the late 1960s and early 1970s for my doctoral work in public health, I personally met with and had discussions regarding these matters with many of the CEOs running such systems. Later, I served as consultant and conceptualizer for the CEOs who started many of the national alliances. Thus, much of the history presented here reflects my personal involvement, as well as my attention and contributions to the literature of the late 1960s and 1970s.) Even in the 1970s there was an expectation that managed care plans would deal with selected groups of providers. Providers recognized this and began to position themselves for this eventuality. Ideas have power even when marketplace realities have not caught up.

While the idea of managed care has been popular, many physicians and hospitals have dreaded its introduction to the market. Networking, mergers, alliances, and the like have been touted as being likely to bring economic and other advantages to managed care systems, but this attitude has obscured the underlying fact that such linkages make managed care more difficult because the system receives bills for service from multiple sources. Nevertheless, networks often have inherent advantages because of the geographic dispersion of member units and the comprehensiveness of their services.

Managed care firms have only recently gained sufficient expertise and market penetration to begin to pressure providers for the efficient care that was anticipated by the pioneers in networks, alliances, and regional hospital systems. Those who prepared early and moved expeditiously are now positioned to benefit from their early efforts to build regional systems. Freestanding hospitals that ignored these trends have found themselves severely handicapped in, if not excluded from, their own marketplaces.

Alliances

Early efforts to develop joint purchasing programs, training, and industrial engineering projects were carried out by trade associations and available to all hospitals. When asked by the public what was being done to contain the rising cost of health care, these programs were trotted out and displayed for all to see. The industry responded to cost concerns through collective programs of purchasing and improvement in the efficiency of individual operations.

By the late 1970s, hospitals had organized national cooperative enterprises like the Voluntary Hospitals of America, SunHealth, Premier Alliance, and American Healthcare Systems to carry out collective enterprises, most notably purchasing. (The major alliances are involved in many other activities, but their central dollar impact and sources of funding come in large part from imposed group purchasing activities.) The national alliances' strategies occurred after HMOs were clearly identified as being able to limit expenditures to hospitals. In addition, the investor-owned hospital groups had gained substantial ground in the marketplace. Unlike state and local hospital associations, alliances were designed to assist their members in gaining competitive advantages over neighboring hospitals. Local competing hospitals were not invited to join. The hospitals forming these national alliances, by and large, tertiary hospitals, but within each alliance complementary hospitals were sought. Within a couple of years after the first major national alliance was started, other alliances formed and began to offer competitive alternatives to hospitals left out of the original alliances. The national level alliances could be described as horizontally integrated, with members of similar character and in non-competing markets. At the local level, each major member set out to build a regional alliance of vertically integrated providers, by securing partners in different geographical areas that would provide referrals to the tertiary hospitals (the hub of the alliance). The national horizontally integrated alliances were built to support the development of local vertically integrated alliances. The national groups provided purchasing (and specialized programmatic resources), while the regional groups worked to build a managed care network configuration.

Were the national alliance efforts at purchasing successful? All of the alliances claim great advantages from such buying cooperatives. Assuming that such programs impact 10 percent of hospital budgets and that group buying reduces prices by 10 percent, this is a 1 percent moderation in costs for all hospitals. While not significant on a yearly basis, compounding such savings over time shows a sizable amount of money ultimately saved.

It is difficult to assess the overall impact of such buying practices. As the hospitals developed oligopolistic buying behavior (by which a few providers affect but do not control the market), the supplier-type companies able to respond grew increasingly few and more powerful. Because the growth rate continues unabated, there is no discernible decline in the growth in health care costs. This makes it difficult to find any consumer benefit coming from this aggregation in the industry. Rebates and price discounts make good public relations copy, so there is little or no complaint about the efficacy of these programs. At a minimum, hospitals have probably gained some clout vis-à-vis powerful national suppliers and moderated prices. These programs represent a modest success in dealing with a modest share of the hospital budget.

Suppliers may have lost a bit of margin in their dealings early on, but probably recouped it later as smaller competitors found it difficult to compete for business with the integrated buyer alliances. With more comprehensive, committed volume contracts, savings are achievable and are probably shared between buyer and seller. Will these advantages squeeze out the small supplier, even when an entrepreneur has a better idea but no access to the large overarching contracts? The story of this aspect of alliances has yet to be told.

The trading of profits and business volumes among firms within the industry has little positive meaning for the consumer. Providers do not usually pass on purchasing savings to consumers. Savings may be retained in the alliance organizations or distributed to the members of the alliance. It makes little difference to the buyers of health services who profits from the vast purchasing power unless the benefits are passed on to consumers. While there is a potential for consumer benefit from the savings realized by alliances, benefits are unlikely because of the price demands buyers of health care services make on provider organizations. With aggregation occurring on the provider side and little buyer pressure for deep price concessions, providers may already have reached a critical mass sufficient to make it possible for them to keep existing prices in place.

Managed Care

Being positioned for survival in a managed care marketplace is the major purpose of national alliances. This is not to say that other purposes were and are not now important. Once institutions are developed, it is well-known that they take on a life of their own and that the "profits" from most such entities, especially those that are not-for-profit, are the benefits that participants derive through participation. Although many of the not-for-profits and cooperatives have developed spin-off operations into for-profit formats that allow executives and members to benefit personally, for the most part the alliances remain not-for-profit enterprises. Executives and compensation experts have long found many ways to

extend equity-type of rewards to the executives so that they operate with many of the same incentives that permeate big business.

Managed care makes it theoretically possible for the most efficient, highest quality providers to win the competition for dedicated blocs of patients and thus become the survivors. In the mid
1970s, when these national alliances were being built, managed
care as we know it today did not exist. It had yet to emerge in most
markets, even though every professional in the health field knew
that the nation had too many hospitals and too many beds (according to American Health Association statistics, there were 1,018,000
hospital beds in service in 1983, and only 887,000 in 1995[8]). In a
fragmented marketplace, managed care firms can induce hospitals and physicians to give discounts to obtain business. But if hospitals merge or are held together in regional networks, few buyers
are able to resist buying from them. Even today, exclusive networks
with full capitation are still only a small part of managed care. Yet,
most of the national and regional alliances represent steps along
the path toward the end they had in mind when they were formed
in the late 1970s.

Managed care plans promise great opportunity for achieving
consumer benefits, but to be successful they require large investments and strong discipline on the part of physicians. Incentives
for physicians to not prescribe drugs or services are at the heart of
medical decision making; they facilitate an efficient system that
offers lower prices due to lower utilization. In some situations, a
regional monopoly or a superior concentration and range of services is needed. In short, success requires highly disciplined physicians committed to reducing the utilization of resources in order
to bring down expenditures so that prices can be lowered for customers. Mere efficiency is not enough, however; purchasers of
health care services must also have sufficient buying power to make
sure that gains in efficiency are passed on to consumers. Neither
theory nor experience indicates that consumers will benefit from
any of these reformations unless buyers are strong and knowledgeable enough to ensure that consumers will share in the benefits of integration.

A number of alliances have tried national managed care ventures with large insurers. Most have failed after years of effort

because members prepared for something for which the market was not yet primed. Readiness depends on individual consumer preference and/or the ability of corporations to channel their employees into a narrow set of choices. As a result, managed care is moving slowly, and a steep learning curve lies ahead. Even the traditional Kaiser-Permanente staff model has problems competing for enrollment because people want free choice. Nevertheless, providers continue to build models that anticipate that consumers' attitudes will change.

Alliances have worked hard to attract additional individual and regional groups of members. A number of systems have chosen to fund and operate regional HMOs that accept risk. Being positioned to offer a network that is geographically dispersed and that offers a comprehensive range of services is of great benefit to major national alliances. Unlike the trade association's purchasing efforts, which were aimed solely at getting a better price per unit purchased, the national alliances' efforts have focused on developing competitive clusters of hospitals in preparation for a managed care world that has not yet arrived.

The record of efforts to build networks to deal with managed care is mixed. In networks built on ownership, it is relatively easy for a cluster of hospitals to deal with managed care firms. But when networks are built on contracts and/or jointly owned organizations, it becomes difficult to bargain over discounted charges that have been set independently by the individual institutions. Most managed care organizations seek large networks and discounted charges, but when the choice of who gets the capitation is among a subset of physician and hospital contracts, such networks may fail, although insurers may benefit. Networks have a hard time attracting volume when hospital members cannot exert sufficient control over personnel and physicians. It challenges credibility to believe that voluntary alliances can make the hard decisions of dropping some physicians and hospitals from existing networks. Even in an owned network, it is nearly impossible to restrict participation to selected physicians. The difficulty in building a network stems from the desire of professionals to keep their practices intact. They avoid change until it becomes essential, and then they attempt to modify the changes to accommodate their own preferred form of practice.

These major fault lines keep most networks in a fragile state, while managed care firms are relatively free to exploit this weakness in alliances.

The difficulty that limited networks have in surviving is akin to the fact that managed care firms also fail. Employers have difficulty getting employee acceptance of limited networks because of the restricted number of providers. Providers likewise resist the constraints of managed care, for reasons similar to those of many consumers.

Hospital organizations that operate regional managed care organizations often find that success has a negative impact. Other managed care organizations resent and react negatively to contracting with hospitals that are their competitors of managed care products and services. When hospitals partner with physicians, they need to appreciate that at some point the physicians will seek opportunities to maximize return on their investment. This expectation of physicians often requires hospitals to sell their managed care plans to competing local managed care organizations that are concerned with gaining market share. In other cases, the success of the hospital organization's managed care plan simply outruns the usefulness and appropriateness of the local hospital's continuing to operate it. In still other situations, the hospital's managed care plan merges with another managed care operation in the region in order to broaden the other operation's ownership and operation of its managed care plan. Even with success, the size, scope, and nature of the managed care plan owned and operated by the hospital often does not match the owner's capability of supporting or growing it. (A colleague related a story to me that highlights some of the difficulties with the buying and selling of physician practices and managed care firms. A local physician group built a successful HMO. They saw themselves as offering a service that made many contributions to the community. When they sold the HMO, they rapidly found that getting a generous price meant that the new owner was interested only in keeping costs down and prices up so as to maximize profits.)

Walston, Kimberly, and Burns[9] raise serious questions about whether hospitals should use ownership as the better mode of relating; instead, they recommend contracting. An integrated network can function effectively only when the incentives of the various parties are aligned. Ownership by itself does not keep the organization functioning smoothly. Some mergers simply do not fit; some groups simply do not make good partners for networks, alliances, or mergers. On the whole, those organizations with heavy investments in assets will continue to pursue the ownership strategy, while insurers will opt for contracting with networks. It is not reasonable to conclude that contractual networks work best for all kinds of participants, either the asset owners or the nonasset owners.

The hospitals and regional systems with the greatest success with managed care are organizations that have strong market share. This makes it possible for them to compete with other managed care organizations without losing business. The market share normally required is substantial, and the hospitals and regional systems also need a reputation among consumers that leads managed care organizations to contract with them in order to attract major business clients for their services. This desire to attract patients is what drives provider strategies as national chains and regional hospital systems continue to seek new members for merger or sale.

National chain organizations have a different history with managed care. The Hospital Corporation of America (HCA) entered into a joint venture with a major insurance company, but the joint venture failed to become a major force in the field. The HCA hospitals' leaders were unable to provide the joint venture any market advantage because the HCA hospitals were not market leaders. Humana (then a hospital company) started its own managed care firm, but ran into substantial resistance to its insurance products from physicians and hospital administrators, who saw their profitability drained away to promote the managed care product. These kinds of difficulties ultimately led Humana to split off the insurance firm from the hospital company, and later to sell the hospital company to another firm, Columbia, which eventually merged with HCA and Health Trust. By 1995, none of the major hospital chains had a strong interest in managed care firms. Their current strategy appears to be to use cost-effectiveness to gain sufficient market share in each regional market so as to become the provider of choice for managed care firms. In addition, they have also built a preferred provider network, Health Advantage. (The importance of preferred provider networks became obvious to me when, at a public hearing, Columbia/HCA was able to say to a prospective joint-venture hospital that they had a network in place with X hospitals and X hundreds of physicians. When their not-for-profit competitor addressed the same issue, all they could say was that a voluntary alliance—members of a national alliance—would build a network, provided that all of the hospitals would agree to do it. Three of their more prominent members had already agreed to be in the Columbia/HCA alliance.)

It is important to note that announced strategies can mask fallback strategies. Provider groups that, because of their substantial market presence (size, geographic dispersion, comprehensiveness), cannot be ignored by managed care firms can, when the market is ready, sell direct to employers.

Future Trends

Given the forces driving the current waves of integration, what seems likely in the next five plus years?

Physicians

The question remains open of how physicians will fit into the overall scenarios envisioned by hospitals and many managed care firms. Physicians are as knowledgeable about the trends as anyone else. Managed care and investor-owned health services are less frightening to physicians than executives of not-for-profit hospitals. Like others, physicians see the consolidation trend and are finding ways to join, control, and/or resist it.

Other trends seem likely to continue. Physicians will continue to form networks for managed care, many of which will be in conjunction with hospitals. However, these forms of affiliation will be relatively weak, with each party continuing to look out for their own individual interest. Additional group practices will form, representing a firmer commitment among physicians to how they will govern themselves and split revenues. Groups have a hefty advantage over alliances and networks. They are a single economic unit, sharing risk, and as long as they do not control a marketplace, they can avoid antitrust problems.

As physicians seek expansion capital and managerial expertise, they will increasingly turn to firms like Caremark, InPhyNet, Phy-

Cor, and Coastal Physician Group, which bring capital and management expertise to the table.[10] The appeal of such firms is that none of them represent hospitals or managed care organizations. They allow physicians to have more input into decisions and to operate as free agents and/or corporate partners when dealing with hospitals and managed care organizations. At some point, these firms are likely to be sold so that the investors can realize gains from building the business. The high bidder may be a hospital, a health care system, or a managed care firm. The reverse might also occur: these firms might end up buying hospitals. Either way, this trend represents the march towards converting physician practices and hospitals into Wall Street–financed businesses.

Insurers

Some of the most dramatic changes have come on the insurance side of health care. Major insurers have been in and out of managed care, with many of the old-line insurers ultimately withdrawing and leaving this niche to firms that deal exclusively with managed care. Blue Cross and Blue Shield plans have made the most impressive turnaround, converting their business from service and indemnity contracts to managed care. These plans have been going through a consolidation phase and now appear fully poised to become equity market firms, which frees them to merge with many other organizations, as well as to tap Wall Street for more equity. Blue Cross and Blue Shield are experimenting with all kinds of integrative moves.

Insurers must build a niche for themselves that deters the efforts of providers to gain sufficient market clout to deal directly with buyers. One avenue is for the insurers to merge with or buy out providers.[11] The key issue is whether this direction is driven by a vision of market protection or by the desire to create a brave new age of efficient care. In any huge firm, the cost of internal transactions can go down, but the tendency to build fiefdoms frustrates this trend and may actually lead to higher costs. Beyond that possibility is the question of competition and monopoly behavior. With fewer competitors in the marketplace there is a danger that provider-insurer entities will use their power to benefit themselves at the expense of the consumers. Getting providers and insurers to be more efficient and price competitive has been a tough job for buyers, even before consolidations occurred. Will it get better with consolidation, or worse? (A recent article in *Fortune* magazine provides a candid description of how price fixing and market allocation works. It portrays sellers as agreeing on market share and price and then moving to bid work in order to achieve these goals. Customers are described as enemies who must be made to pay to keep up prices and sellers' profits.)[12] As providers seek legislation to permit market consolidations that go beyond current antitrust guidelines, they are seeking to be the community guardians of supply and price. Because they did not undertake reform in the past, the ceding of such powers is risky. Recent history suggests that providers continue to resist changing their ways, and both managed care firms and insurers can be expected to resist unless they are part of the deal.

Academic Medical Centers

Academic medical centers have been at the tail end of the parade. However, investor-owned chains are now looking for economic ties to such centers of excellence. If an organization seeks to be the regional provider of choice, then these academic institutions need to be part of the effort. The Mayo Clinic recognized this necessity and moved to develop national and regional satellites. Teaching centers are now reaching out in ways unheard of five years ago. Some academic centers have joined Columbia/HCA in markets where the academic medical center completes the regional, full-service package of services. In the future, more alliances can be expected as not-for-profit hospital systems seek to link up as a competitive response to the investor-owned market.

Community Hospitals

Community hospitals will continue to merge with regional players, including investor-owned chains. No hospital believes that it can remain outside and independent when the dominate belief is that buyers will choose networks. Networks will choose to send business to their own hospitals rather than to affiliated hospitals. Sophisticated buyer groups might select such hospitals, but providers have ten years of system experience and buyers are just beginning to consider purchasing coalitions. Sellers of services are bundling their activities, while buyers (including managed care firms) are seeking to unbundle, resulting in a tug of war that will continue for the near term.

Regional Multihospital Health Systems

Regional multihospital health systems are the organizations best positioned to become the providers of choice for managed care or direct contracting. They will continue to bring more and more physicians (especially in primary care) into the fold. The most extensive elaboration of this model is in Minneapolis, where three or four systems have already integrated physicians and managed care. This integration has led to employer uneasiness about concentration and pricing. These employers are concerned with how to break through the domination by provider-insurer conglomerates in order to achieve greater efficiencies than are currently available. In Missouri, the regional hospital system to watch is BJC, an entity formed from Barnes, Jewish, Christian, Baptist, and a variety of other hospitals in the region.

While a number of these systems have secured ownership consolidation, they have become captives to the status quo and have not achieved anywhere near the efficiencies anticipated by the industry watchers. Incorporation of different cultures has been a problem, as has the reduction of consumer choice.

In the near term, additional mergers of single hospitals into systems can be anticipated. Systems also will merge, and a growing number of them will sell to insurers. Conversely, insurers can be expected to build networks through contractual relationships. They will avoid acquisitions until prices for such operations are lower. Prices will come down as hospitals are forced to compete on price. Mergers of hospitals in smaller markets will lower the cost for technology and overhead, but by doing so, they will eliminate price competition.

Overall Prognosis

The health field's anticipation of managed care and fear of investor-owned hospital chains continues to drive consolidations, which will continue into the indefinite future. Before physicians become fully integrated into managed care, they will go through intermediary forms, including group practice and becoming units of national firms, employees of managed care firms, and employees of hospitals. These intermediary forms of ownership make it possible for physicians to increase the value of their business. A well-balanced group of primary and specialty physicians has a greater value than would the same number of solo physicians.

What is occurring is an incremental, disjointed movement toward new forms of health care organization. Two forces are at work, one defensive and protective, the other entrepreneurial. Managed care plans, investor-owned hospital chains, physician group practices, and other forms of collaboration are putting pressure on the health care system. Traditional health care organizations are modifying themselves to compete. Networks and systems are concerned with improving coordination by allocating resources to those points that advantage the system. Coordinating roles and activities in a system takes power and influence away from the traditional units. New systems are becoming the centers of power. Those systems that best master the new roles that are emerging will become the new leaders in the health care field. Some will come from traditional positions, but others will come from outside the field. What proportion comes from each source will depend on who masters the new technologies needed to make integrated systems work.

As the field consolidates, the future will be even more complex. There is a real possibility that a handful of national firms will eventually dominate health care, but the route to that end is two steps forward, three back, and forward again. The partners for the dance are still shifting. (As I was finishing the first draft of this paper, I received a copy of a conference report by Arnold D. Kaluzny, Howard S. Zuckerman, and Thomas C. Ricketts III.[13] It is an excellent source of thought on the performance and structure of alliances. While many of the authors of the conference papers are already adequately cited in this chapter's notes, the report represents the latest thinking on the important issues related to health care.)

Notes

1. A collection of earlier papers on this subject is contained in Brown, M. (Ed.). *Strategy and Structures in Health Care Management, A Best-of-*

Health-Care-Management-Review Publication. Frederick, Md.: Aspen, 1992.

2. "AmHS, Premier Alliances to Merge." *Modern Healthcare,* August 7, 1995, pp. 2–3.

3. Zuckerman, H. S., Kaluzny, A. D., and Ricketts, T. C. "Alliances in Health Care: What We Know, What We Think We Know, and What We Should Know." *Health Care Management Review,* 1995, *20*(1), 54–64.

4. Shortell, S. M. "The Evolution of Hospital Systems: Unfulfilled Promises and Self-Fulfilling Prophesies." *Medical Care Review,* 1988, *45*(2), 177–214.

5. Brown, M., and Nickles, P. J. "Court Shoots Down Antitrust Immunity." *Modern Healthcare,* August 1982, pp. 164–168.

6. Nickles, P. J., Tucker, G., and Brown, M. "Analysis Probes Risk of Antitrust Suit." *Modern Healthcare,* December 1982, pp. 104–109.

7. Brown, M., and others. "Trends in Multihospital Systems: A Multiyear Comparison." *Health Care Management Review,* 1980, *5*(4), 9–22.

8. "AHA Statistics." *Economic Trends,* 1996, *11*(1).

9. Walston, S. L., Kimberly, J. R., and Burns, L. R. "Vertical Integration in Health Care." *Health Care Management Review,* 1995, *21*(1), 83–92.

10. "Doc Practice Management Set to Explode." *Modern Healthcare,* August 14, 1995, pp. 26–31.

11. For a more detailed examination of some of the issues involved here, see Wolford, R., Brown, M., and McCool, B. "Getting to Go in Managed Care." *Health Care Management Review,* 1993, *18*(1), 7–20.

12. "My Life as a Corporate Mole for the FBI." *Fortune,* September 4, 1995, pp. 52–62. For a more complete discussion of some of these issues, see Nguyen, N. X. "Hospital Markets and Competition: Implications for Antitrust Policy." *Health Care Management Review,* 1994, *19*(1), 34–44.

13. Kaluzny, A. D., Zuckerman, H. S., and Ricketts, T. C., III. *Partners For the Dance: Forming Strategic Alliances in Health Care.* Ann Arbor, Mich: Health Administration Press, 1995.

Chapter Three

Public Trust in America's Hospitals

Everett A. Johnson
Richard L. Johnson

When the question of the public's trust in hospitals is viewed from the perspective of growth in diagnostic and therapeutic capabilities, the hospital has never stood higher in public opinion. Citizens are proud of their hospitals and what their hospitals can do to alleviate pain and suffering. At the same time, people are resentful of the costs of health care and afraid of being hospitalized with inadequate coverage, or none at all. In today's world, the decision to change jobs may depend on whether or not one will be covered for health care benefits.

The paradox is a fascinating one, because U.S. patients can receive the very best care available in the world but lose their life savings in the process. Most of the health care systems in other developed countries hold the U.S. hospitals and medical care in high regard, as something to which they aspire. Other countries' libraries routinely receive the leading medical and hospital journals from the United States. Clearly, there is much to admire in our health system.

However, there is much to be concerned about when the costs of health care are examined. For decades, the annual expenditure increases for health care in the United States have exceeded the national rate of inflation. It is routinely reported that health care expenditures in the United States constitute a higher percentage (now exceeding 14 percent) of the gross domestic product (GDP) than in any other country. To demonstrate why the American public has lost trust in hospitals requires dealing with health care expenditures. Conversely, to demonstrate why the American public continues to have confidence in hospitals requires pointing to the diagnostic and therapeutic accomplishments of the past several decades. A great deal of evidence can be marshaled in support of either position.

Probing beneath the surface, the question of public trust in hospitals is much more complicated, however, and not resolvable by the present system. In 1948, during the Truman administration, a serious effort was made to create a national health service with the introduction in Congress of the Wagner, Murray, Dingell bill. The entitlement program proposed by this bill was believed to be a program whose time had come. In retrospect, it turned out to be a program whose time had not come; Congress couldn't get enough votes to pass it. The question lying behind the issue of public trust today is not the same question as it was then. The question today is, What major restructuring of the health field is needed to provide access to all persons at a "reasonable" cost? Reasonable cost is defined as restraining expenditures for health care services to more modest levels, using the annual inflation rate as the guidepost. The funds for broadening access would be obtained from a combination of federal funding, new legislation requiring prepayment organizations to accept all who apply, standardized and simplified reporting of claims, and greater hospital efficiencies. The question of public trust will turn on finding answers that have been elusive for nearly half a century.

From the standpoint of the public, four questions need to be answered:

1. How is access for all of the population to be assured?
2. How can health care costs be restrained to reasonable levels?
3. What sources of funding can be used to assure access to the health care system?
4. What steps can be taken to make the health care system efficient?

Of little concern to the public is whether or not these four questions might lead to the bankruptcy of the health care system. A look at the way government has behaved in the past may provide some insights into what providers can expect in the future.

Historical Insights

When Titles XVIII and XIX (Medicare and Medicaid) were enacted in the early 1960s, the federal government embarked on a
new road by paying for care on an age-related segment of the population and for the economically disadvantaged. At the time these
programs commenced, beneficiaries received units of service and
hospitals were paid audited costs. Dollars were applied to the units
of service to determine the amount to be paid to providers. The
federal government quickly learned that this approach had two
built-in difficulties. As the cost per unit of service increased, federal dollars had to increase. The government also discovered that
the number of budgeted units of service was too low and the number of services exceeded government estimates. Year after year,
total costs of the program rose steadily. Two decades later, expenses
are still increasing, as shown in Table 3.1.

By 1980, there was general agreement that Medicare expenditure increases had to be moderated. To slow the use of Medicare,
diagnosis-related groups (DRGs) were adopted in 1983 as the
method of payment. A fixed dollar amount was paid for each
Medicare admission, and the number of days of care and the hospital services utilized per admission were no longer used as measures. To adjust for yearly inflation, Congress included a formula
that relied on changes in the medical market basket component
of the GDP. It did not take long for the federal government to back
away from this formula without actually repealing the section in
the legislation that had established it. Instead, the Health Care
Financing Administration (HCFA) utilized back-door methods to
annually restrict payments to hospitals to less than what was called
for in the legislation.

Several years of restricted payments have taken their toll.
Medicare now pays somewhat less than operating cost to hospitals,
and Medicaid pays substantially less. To compensate for these
shortfalls, hospitals have increasingly engaged in cost shifting by
inflating billed charges to other categories of patients. This practice has reached the point where patients receiving their bills following discharge undergo "sticker shock" of major proportions,
which has led many members of the public to view both hospitals
and physicians as greedy and not to be trusted. It does no good for

Table 3.1. National Health Care Expenditures, 1970–1990.

Year	Number of Persons 65 and Older[1]	Total Health Care Expenditures[1]	Medicare Expenditures[2]	Percentage Increase in Medicare Expenditures[2]	Medicare Expenditure as a Percentage of Total Health Expense[2]
1970	19.9M	$74.4B	$7.6B	—	10.2 percent
1980	25.5M	$250.1B	$37.5B	393 percent	15.0 percent
1990	31.1M	$666.2B	$111.2B	196 percent	16.7 percent

[1]*Source:* U.S. Bureau of the Census, *Statistical Abstract of the United States: 1992* (112th ed.). Washington, D.C.: Department of Commerce, 1992, Table 12, "Total Population, by Age and Sex: 1980 to 1991."

[2]*Source:* U.S. Bureau of the Census, *Statistical Abstract of the United States: 1992* (112th ed.). Washington, D.C.: Department of Commerce, 1992, Table 135, "National Health Expenditures: 1960 to 1990."

hospitals to blame the federal government for this situation when patients query the hospital about their bills. Whether this explanation is true or not, the public is not accepting it; rather, people are concluding that they are being treated unfairly, and they resent the hospital, not the federal government.

At the turn of the twentieth century, hospitals were far different institutions than they are in the closing decade of the century. Because at the turn of the century there were few diagnostic and therapeutic services, nursing care was the dominant hospital role. Religious groups undertook to provide havens for those who were ill. Emotional support was given by nurses dedicated to serving humanity by providing tender loving care. Nursing was a calling, not a career. Hospital corridors were the domain of "angels of mercy."

Slowly, but at an ever quickening pace following World War II, technology forged toward the forefront, until today it is the driving force in the modern hospital. If a nurse from the year 1900 were transported into today's hospital, she would have difficulty recognizing it as a hospital. In all probability, the equipment now available in profusion would lead her to conclude that she was in a technological institute. This nurse would not understand the concept of DNR (do not resuscitate). What was a charitable or public institution for the ill has turned into a technological marvel. The ability to do good has been replaced with the ability to do well.

The Changing Role of Hospitals

As the primary measure of judging hospitals, "doing well" has led to profound changes in society's expectations about health care. A comparison of 1950 to 1990, a period of 40 years, shown in Table 3.2, demonstrates what has taken place.

Had hospitals continued to operate as they did in 1950, the population increase of 64.1 percent would have led to a total of 11,132 hospitals in 1990 and hospitals would be operating 1.989 million beds. What happened instead was a decline of 2.0 percent in the number of hospitals and a 15.5 percent decline in the number of beds. Even though the population increased by nearly two thirds, the number of inpatient admissions rose by 80 percent. The public's use of hospitals increased even more dramatically, with outpatient visits more than doubling since 1973. Surgery, which in

Table 3.2. Selected National Hospital Data, 1950–1990.

Factor	1950	1990	Percentage of Change
U.S. population[1]	152.27M	249.92M	+64.1 percent
Number of hospitals[2]	6,788	6,649	−2.0 percent
Number of beds	1.436M	1.213M	−15.5 percent
Inpatient admissions	18.48M	33.77M	+82.0 percent
Outpatient visits[3]	181.37M	368.18M	+103.0 percent
Full-time employees	1.058M	4.063M	+284.0 percent
Total expenses	$3.65B	$234.87B	+6,435 percent

[1]*Source:* U.S. Bureau of the Census. *Statistical Abstract of the United States: 1992* (112th ed.). Washington, D.C.: Department of Commerce, 1992, p. 6, Table 1.

[2]*Source:* American Hospital Association. *Hospital Statistics: 1991–92.* Chicago, Ill: American Hospital Association, 1991, Table 1.

[3]American Hospital Association, *Hospital Statistics: 1970.* Chicago, Ill: American Hospital Association, 1970, Table 1.

1990 was divided evenly between ambulatory and inpatient, was all inpatient in 1950.

To accommodate these changes, the number of full-time employees of these developing technological institutes also grew, not by the same two-thirds as the population, but by nearly four-and-one-half times. The shift that has taken place is best seen in the costs of hospital care: over the forty-year period, total expenses increased by 6,435 percent (from $3.65 billion to $234.8 billion).

Looking back over the twentieth century in light of these statistics is instructive. In 1900, hospitals were a low-cost industry employing cheap labor, thanks to the work of many religious groups. By 1990, hospitals had become highly labor and capital intensive. Unlike nearly all other forms of organization, hospitals have found themselves unable to substitute capital for labor, or vice versa. Instead, capital and labor have been additive, with the result being skyrocketing costs. As hospitals have become more technologically sophisticated, unskilled positions have been upgraded and workers replaced with higher-paid skilled personnel.

Hospitals were not the only health care providers to succumb to technology. In 1900, the family doctor had spent four years in medical school and one year in internship, and made house calls carrying his little black bag, only to be replaced with an army of skilled physician specialists who have spent seven to ten years learning their profession. Health care is now a costly matter to those who provide the services, as well as to those who use these services.

Health care is a troubling issue in our society because it is not amenable to solutions that are applied successfully in other industries. As technological enterprises, hospitals are driven by the escalation of costs. Medical staffs want a hospital to install the latest and newest equipment, and they will continue to push for it. Salaries for scarce personnel continue to outpace the rate of inflation. Competition among these technological enterprises continues unabated in local communities, in spite of all the protests that such head-to-head competition serves no useful purpose.

As long as competition among hospitals continues, cost containment programs will not be successful. The cost-control program of the Nixon administration failed, as did the voluntary cost-containment program sponsored by the American Hospital Association in the 1980s. Even the state-controlled Certificate of Need (CON) laws have failed to control hospitals' capital expenditures. Two-fifths of the states have abandoned CON programs in the last forty years, resulting in an increase in the public's trust in the outcomes of hospitalization; but it has also led to a distrust in the costs of care, and regulations to restrict those costs.

Regulation Versus Marketplace Realities

Today, a myriad of regulatory restrictions to health care prohibit providers from applying sound marketing principles to offset competitive threats to institutional survival. Examples of these efforts and their effects on hospitals are shown in Table 3.3.

Hospitals are now faced with a Congress and administration determined to rein in hospital costs and provide access to health care for those who are uninsured, and to accomplish these goals without adding to the federal fiscal deficit. Concerns being raised by providers about endangering quality of care or about the likelihood of bankruptcy are not apt to be heard, or they may simply be dismissed as hospitals crying wolf in the present climate, in which further marketplace restrictions are likely.

Historically, health insurance premiums have been tax deductible for companies, no matter what the extent of the employee

Table 3.3. Hospital Responses to
Regulatory Restrictions on Health Care.

Regulation	Regulator Viewpoint	Hospital Viewpoint
Fraud and abuse regulations	Protect the patient and the federal government.	Interfere with the extent and variety of incentives for higher productivity.
Certificate of Need programs	Control unnecessary building programs.	Interfere with sound economic/social programming and restrict the ability of a hospital to compete with other health care providers.
Antitrust rules	Economically protect the patient from financial abuse.	Increase the cost of health care.
Rate regulation	Protects the public (in four states).	Interferes with hospitals keeping up-to-date in technology.
Programming regulations	Incremental increases in programs can be financed piecemeal or hidden in existing funding.	Programming has to be tied explicitly to specific funding.
Medicare regulations	Total dollars of Medicare outlay must be constrained.	Medicare outlays should increase to accommodate additional enrollees, and absence of inflation adjustments in Medicare payments threatens bankruptcy.
Regulations in general	Primary concern is meeting one-year budget goals.	Primary concern is long-term survival.

benefits provided. Employees with extensive health care benefits are treated, taxwise, the same as employees who are covered by programs with minimal benefits. Congressional conflict arises over the question of whether health benefits are primarily a tax issue or a health care concern. Treated as a tax, there is inequity, but viewed as health policy, more comprehensive protection is better, from a social policy perspective. The debate is unclear as to whether increased availability of health care benefits or a reduction in the federal deficit is more important.

The pressures on Congress suggest that any major change in health care is going to have to be financed through increased efficiency gains, new sources of revenue, or a decrease in the use of the health care resources. Federal legislators are well aware that the pressing economic issues of today preclude a costly increase in government spending for health services to the uninsured. This attitude is understandable when Congressional concerns are reviewed:

- A federal deficit requiring $200 billion annually to service the debt
- Persistent trade imbalances due to global competition with U.S. products
- Strong public sentiment against increasing taxes, unless such funds are used to decrease the deficit
- A strong military posture as international policeman
- Continuing efforts to control inflation
- A desire to expand social programs to cover disadvantaged groups

In the face of these major problems, a miscalculation about the costs of substantial changes in access and use of the health care system could have serious consequences for the economic health of the nation. For Congress to undertake a restructuring of the health field would require belief in the following assumptions:

1. The exercise of central authority and control by a federal agency can effectively moderate spending by health care providers.
2. A central authority can determine wisely and prudently the allocation of health care resources within the various parts of the system.

3. Expenditures for health care can be harmonized with the availability of funds.
4. Centralized control over health care expenditures is essential to moving toward a balanced federal budget.

In the event that these assumptions turn out to be overly ambitious, the outcome will not be known until the new, restructured health care plan is in place and operational for one to two years. Therefore, before enacting changes in the health care system, a key question needs to be examined that does not appear to be on any agenda: What happens to the providers of care if all efforts to moderate increases in health care expenditures are ineffective? As yet, there is not much interest in examining this possibility. Instead, glib statements are offered by various advocates of change that a uniform simple billing form, reform of tort laws, community rating instead of experience rating, defining outcome measures of medical care, and other overgeneralized statements will serve to address the cost issues satisfactorily. There is a strong belief among those advocating major change that health care costs can become "reasonable." Buttressing their position is a corollary belief that corporate America will no longer permit the type of cost escalations that have been taking place. Yet, all hospitals, not just a few, are both labor and capital intensive. What happens to one hospital's budget also happens to the budgets of other hospitals in the community. Though there may be some differences among local hospitals' costs from year to year, the same upward trend exists for all.

In the short run, a corporation may exercise its market power in selecting its hospital provider, but it must be careful not to drive competing hospitals out of business or it may restrict its own care options in the future. When corporations reach a point in negotiations with hospitals where prices are firm and hospitals are unwilling to negotiate further, corporations will have to resort to more traditional methods for limiting future premium increases. They will have to increase deductibles and co-payments, cap maximum payments, restrict services, or find other ways of reducing corporate exposure by passing on the additional costs to employees.

Corporate executives who sit on local hospital boards of directors annually approve institutional budgets. By approving a hospital budget, board members are signifying approval of any increases

in expense or revenue. In doing so, they are agreeing with the rationale on which a budget is based. Corporate executives as hospital
directors vote for the best interests of the institution, even though
the next time they sit down with their employee benefits manager
to discuss next year's health insurance premium, they may feel quite
differently. This is not a contradiction, but rather a recognition that
what makes good sense in one setting may make for difficulties in
another setting. In this type of situation, the corporate execu-
tive/hospital director devotes his efforts to solving the corporate
problem, and leaves the solving of the health care problem to someone else, presumably government. Once again, the public's trust is
abused because the basic issue is not being confronted.

Achieving Reasonable Costs

With hospitals both labor and capital intensive, is it possible to
achieve "reasonable" health care costs? In examining the possibilities, three categories are often identified as needing attention: hospitals, physicians, and third-party payers. With respect to hospitals,
the ongoing changes frequently noted are

- Patient-focused care
- Total quality improvement programs
- Productivity improvement
- Capitation of hospital fees as a replacement for DRGs
- Development of systems
- Strict limitations on "safe harbors"
- Adoption of managed care for Medicare

For physicians, the list of changes includes

- Resource-based relative value scales
- Stricter government requirements for determining fraud and
  abuse
- Increased number of primary care physicians
- Growth in multispecialty group practices

For third-party payers, the list includes

- Expansion of managed care
- Adoption of community rating
- Creation of a uniform, simplified claims system

On the surface, this formidable list seems to include all the elements needed to accomplish the goal of restraining health care cost increases. However, it does not reflect several important factors that are affecting and will affect efforts to control health care costs:

- An aging population (over seventy-five years) that is now 13 percent of the total population
- An age cohort of seventy-five years and up that will grow by 3.5 million persons by 2000 A.D. and that uses health care at eight times the rate of those sixty-five and younger
- An inflation factor that is expected to run at 4 to 5 percent annually for the rest of the decade
- A physician population that will reach 2.45 per 1,000 population by 2000 A.D.
- Interest rates that will rise and increase the cost of carrying the national debt
- Continued investments by hospitals in new technology, probably at an increasing rate
- Redesign and construction of hospitals to accommodate the growth of ambulatory care
- Hiring of highly skilled and therefore more expensive personnel to operate more sophisticated equipment
- Hiring of more experienced and diversified management talent
- Continued enforcement of antitrust laws

If this list outweighs the previous list of "reasonable" changes, and suggests that strong, upward pressures for increasing health care costs will continue, then the controls put in place by Congress to restrict expenditures will have to operate successfully. If they are to do so, hard decisions will be required of the federal government. To establish limits on health care expenditures, steps may be required that shelve technological advances, restrict salary increases, limit access by permitting long queues, and accept poorer levels of quality, all in the interest of maintaining absolute control over the elements of cost.

Faced with the necessity for making such decisions, the question of how the American public might react needs to be considered. Will they accept poorer quality service and long waiting times—for instance, up to three months for an operation? Examples of inadequate funding in other fields include public education, which has been allowed to deteriorate when there has been a choice between higher local taxes or loss in quality of the educational system. Negative changes in both areas have been accepted by the public and have not led to a sustained public outcry. Will the same hold true for health care if the same type of choice is made? It might turn out that the public is more seriously concerned about deterioration in the health care system. Changes that will affect health, or life and death matters, are likely to have more personal implications and to hit closer to home than changes to education, and might thus be regarded in a different light by the general public.

The significance of such a choice in health care is more serious in another sense as well. If hospital services have to deteriorate in order for hospitals to survive financially, will physicians accept limitations on their ordering of hospital diagnostic or treatment modalities? At the margins—that is, in decision making that may or may not affect the patient's care, such as whether to provide an EKG for a heart patient every day or only every other day—will physicians accept such limitations or will they take the position that it is the hospital's responsibility to find the necessary funds to keep services up-to-date? A miscalculation in the enactment of legislation would be costly, and further imbalance the federal budget. By not addressing this possibility up front, a serious risk is run if, for example, a program to increase accessibility is put in place and then a serious miscalculation is discovered. There will be no turning back; reversing legislation will not be an alternative, nor will continuing with the new program be an option. The result of such a situation will be a further decrease in public trust in both the hospital and the political process.

As a society, Americans do not readily accept governmental dictates, and when they find regulations onerous, they look for ways around them. The United States is only one of two nations with a predominately private health care system (South Africa is the other), and any new federal program needs to be concerned with what hospitals and physicians might do if public financing became too restrictive. In undertaking a restructuring of health care, caution must be exercised to avoid taking the brakes off the public's use of the health care system. At the moment, the public is most concerned about the costs of health care, while politicians are concerned with accessibility as well as costs. Providers could conclude that the public places a high value on hospital services and wants to be assured that they can receive care when needed, no matter what their personal economic situation.

Global Budgeting

With the inauguration of the Clinton administration, new words were introduced to describe a concept for limiting health care expenditures: *global budgeting*. Although the term was new, the concept is a variation of the cost controls of the Nixon years and the cost containment efforts of the Reagan years. Global budgeting envisions caps on expenditures for health care providers, but the financing of care remains pluralistic, with both government and private sources utilized. The government might establish a requirement that carriers provide a minimum package of health care benefits, which could be exceeded by purchasing additional benefits or amenities through the commercial market, and payments to providers could be higher as long as minimum standards are met.

To adopt global budgeting for expenditures but not for payment to providers would permit "gaming the system"—that is, private carriers that would pay higher amounts to providers would be preferred by both hospitals and physicians striving to maximize revenue because expenditure caps could not be exceeded. Patients covered by public funding sources would not be the preferred category of patient. Hospitals that regard themselves as technological enterprises that need to stay on the cutting edge of medical advances would take whatever steps were necessary to allow them to remain the best.

The only way to avoid preferential treatment under a global budget is for payment schedules to providers to be identical for both private and publicly financed care, thus eliminating windfalls for those providers who could skim off the better-paying patients. The idea of one payment schedule for all, coupled with a global budget on expenditures, suggests that there would no longer be a need for a combination of public and private financing—only one agency would be needed. Such a conclusion opens the door for a national health program.

Assuming that global budgeting is directed only at expenditures by health care providers, the political reality of increasing access for the 38 million persons currently uninsured needs to be addressed. The number of uninsured represents 15 percent of the population. Granted, they do receive some care, to an extent that has not been quantified; but if access were to be provided on a formalized basis and counted, a 15 percent increase would occur and would have to be taken into account in a global budget.

Hospital costs can be expected to increase by a minimum of 79 percent from 1991 to 2001 due to three factors completely outside the ability of hospitals to control: (1) access will need to be provided to the additional previously uninsured 15 percent of the population; (2) growth of the seventy-five years and older age cohort and of the under-sixty-five cohort will account for another 16 percent impact on health care expenditures; (3) inflation, if it increases annually an average of 4 percent, will push costs up by 48 percent. This total projected 79 percent increase does not include additional increases for technology improvements or other factors that may have to be considered. In the face of a $4.4 trillion national deficit, an increase in health care costs of this magnitude would further jar the public's trust.

If in restructuring the health care field the government mandates underwriting on a community rating basis rather than on an experience rating basis, they will create a difficult problem of enforcement for themselves. Agreeing that community rating is desirable is a very different matter than making sure that it is effective in operation. Avoiding adverse selection will be as important to a carrier under community rating as it is under experience rating. Even if social equity were to be mandated, prepayment organizations would continue to be concerned primarily with their own financial viability. Finding ways to appear to be living with community rating but at the same time not disadvantaging themselves in the competitive marketplace will become a major concern for carriers.

Capitating Hospital Fees

A strategy now appearing on the horizon is the notion that hospital fees should be capitated for patients covered by public funding. This is the next step in shifting financial risk from the federal government to hospitals. When Medicare and Medicaid programs were enacted, the government's position was for hospitals to provide the care and the government to provide the financing. Hospitals were paid a per diem rate based on their costs, adjusted for the area of the country and the degree of urbanization. When the government reviewed its expenditures fifteen years later, it concluded that it was spending too much money, so in 1983 it adopted the DRG program. Rather than pay for the cost of each day of care, the federal government unilaterally shifted to paying a stipulated amount for each admission. There was no negotiation with hospitals for the amount to be paid per admission because the government was already paying for more than 40 percent of the total inpatient days of care in acute hospitals. Rates simply were announced in the *Federal Register.* As in the cost-based system of payment, the number of admissions paid for under DRGs has now outstripped available funds.

If capitated rates are adopted as the method of payment by the federal government, stability of funding will be achieved by shifting the control of units of service to hospitals. Unfortunately, hospitals do not control admissions or discharges; these are a function of physicians, who make these decisions based on clinical necessity and not on their financial impact on hospitals. If capitated rates were enacted, it is to be expected that they would not be a subject of negotiation between an individual hospital and the government, but rather would appear once again in the *Federal Register* as an accomplished fact. Resorting to this formula for payment would not only protect the federal government's budget, it would at the same time leave existing benefits in place. Congress would not have to take any heat that might come from public reaction to use of this approach.

Up to the present, national health policy has been developed on an incremental basis. As a result, it is implicit, inconsistent, and contradictory. Under the Prospective Payment System—by which the government pays a lump sum to hospitals for each of 411 categories of illness, the amount varying depending on the location of the hospital and the intensity of the illness—the pattern of policy making has been piecemeal. Table 3.4 illustrates the pattern of implicit congressional policies, the problems faced by the providers, and the consequences of the policies.

Looking Ahead

A look ahead to the year 2000 could provide some insights into the potential impact of a major restructuring of the health care system. An understanding of what might happen will permit an evaluation of the validity of assumptions already made at the federal level.

Congress appears to be thinking that the existing programs of Medicare and Medicaid should be continued and that access to them should be expanded, but at the same time, that dollars to providers should be more stringently limited. The inescapable conclusion is that this equation simply cannot be made to work. Two outcomes can be foreseen. First, if access to health care benefits is to be provided to all citizens, the federal government will be required to increase expenditures for health care. Financing of access for everyone has to come from more sources than increased efficiency in hospital operations. Second, if federal dollars for health care turn out to be inadequate, one of the two following sets of conditions will ensue: (1) the federal government will redefine its responsibilities in health care and adopt a more modest role, in keeping with a limited ability to finance its commitments; or (2) the legitimate financial interests of hospitals will go unrecognized until there are significant institutional bankruptcies and patient care is denied to federally sponsored individuals.

What can be done? Although an all-inclusive health care policy that wraps all of the existing problems into one elegant solution is desirable, it nevertheless is a financially risky undertaking at a time when there is significant public pressure to reduce the national deficit. Because the federal establishment has no direct responsibility for providing patient care to the general public, it is

Table 3.4. Congressional Patterns of Policy Making.

Implicit/Explicit Policy	Providers' Problems	Consequences to Providers
1. Access for everyone	Inadequate financing	Mission vs. margin (profits)/irrational hospital closures
2. Coverage for the uninsured	Closing emergency rooms Increasing bad debts	Providers at risk
3. Coverage for the underinsured	Employers move employees from full-time to part-time	No coverage to pay bills
4. Expansion of Medicare to nonacute care (drugs, etc.)	Recipients don't understand coverage limitation and blame hospitals	Revenues decreasing at a faster rate than costs
5. Acceptable quality of care to all citizens	Lack of definition of quality of care	Increase in lawsuits
6. Part B payments are out of control and need to be controlled	Increase in number of physicians refusing to care for Medicare patients	Limited access
7. Increasing Medicare enrollment funded out of existing funds	Developing greater productivity Finding offsetting sources of revenue Restricting salary increases	Increase in transfers to public hospitals Other carriers refuse to permit cost shifting Loss of personnel

likely to give first priority to the needs of the federal budget. Any shortfalls due to underfunding of mandated benefits by health care programs will first come out of hospital budgets and only belatedly out of federal funds. Striving to create a "once and for all" program that properly aligns all of the characteristics of the complex, technological health care industry is a task of immense proportions. Hospitals are dynamic, changing, and in flux; what was true yesterday is no longer true today, and will change again tomorrow. Such rapid changes make it very difficult to develop a health care policy that serves all of the public interests for the foreseeable future. Yet, a new federal policy is urgently needed. To be successful, such a policy must fit within the budgetary constraints of government, while at the same time placing on the health care system no financial demands that cannot be met.

Two questions need to be answered when seeking new solutions to the health care cost dilemma: (1) What is the appropriate role for the federal government in keeping with its ability to fund health care? and (2) What steps can the federal government take to encourage a free market response to health care needs not funded by the federal government? Table 3.5 presents a conceptual framework for thinking about these two questions.

If the dynamic changes occurring in the health care field are permitted to continue, it will be necessary to avoid a centralized control that will

1. Lock the status quo into place
2. Greatly inhibit organizational modifications
3. Prevent shifts in the use of resources
4. Reduce advances in medical technology

At the same time, it will be unreasonable to leave health care in the hands of an unrestricted free marketplace. A mix of government and the free market is needed. Certain principles need to be agreed upon if both government and hospitals are to regain public trust.

1. Health care is best provided when it is responsive at the local level, which requires decisions to be made at that level. Two basic practices dictate the local nature of health care:
   a. When individuals become sick, they seek the emotional support of family members. If hospitalized, they prefer a local hospital, for the convenience of the family.
   b. Attending physicians prefer to call upon local consultants or to refer to local physicians if they are serving as a primary care physician, because referrals are informal and highly subjective.

Table 3.5. A Conceptual Framework for Thinking About the Government Role in Controlling Health Care Costs.

Type of Coverage	Benefits	Financing Mechanism	Eligibility	Providers
Mandated	Catastrophic coverage	SSA (individual contributions)	Mandated for employed persons Voluntary enrollment	Acute care hospitals Physicians
Free market	Elective coverage	Third-party payers Commercial Blue Cross HMO PPO Self-pay	Determined by coverage	Free choice or determined by coverage
Mandated minimum standards	Mandated minimum coverage	Voucher Government purchase Free market purchase	Third-party payers Licensed	Free choice or determined by coverage

2. The federal government's responsibility is to establish a ceiling for individual health care costs beyond which a national catastrophic coverage program would assume the expenses.
3. For persons who cannot afford or who are unable to obtain coverage, the federal government should provide a voucher to be used to purchase coverage for basic benefits from a provider.
4. The free market should be allowed to operate below the level of catastrophic coverage, with the exception of those categories of disadvantaged citizens who are provided a voucher.

Elements of a Successful National Health Care Policy

The basic building block for a national health care policy should be *public entitlement* to catastrophic coverage to avoid bankruptcy as the result of an illness, either acute or chronic. Eligibility for participation must be open to the self-employed, nonworking persons, students, employees, and retirees—all persons in the country, regardless of their social or financial well-being. The second fundamental element of success would be a *minimum level of coverage* for every citizen. Organizations that wanted to compete in the free marketplace would be certified to ensure that they offered benefits equal or superior to the established minimum standards. To the disadvantaged and those unable to pay, the government (preferably at the federal level) would issue vouchers to be used to purchase minimum coverage in the recipient's local domain.

Principles of Catastrophic Coverage

While minimum benefits pay only a limited amount per day, in spite of the actual costs (for example, $300, although the cost may be $800), catastrophic coverage pays for everything beyond a certain dollar amount (such as everything over $1,000). In planning for catastrophic coverage, four basic principles should be followed:

1. Create a normal distribution curve by covering as many people as possible.
2. Commence coverage at a dollar level that is high enough to support a modest monthly premium.

3. Provide coverage only for acute care in hospitals, but pay all associated hospital costs and professional fees.
4. Provide a simple way to pay premiums for coverage.

Catastrophic coverage should be designated for the general public, not for only a segment of the population. From a statistical standpoint, the worst possible choice would be to provide catastrophic coverage only for people aged sixty-five and older, the Medicare enrollees. This segment of the population (the cohort of those sixty-five to seventy-four and the cohort of those seventy-five and older) makes the greatest use of hospital resources, consuming hospital care at a rate five times that of under-sixty-five cohort, a situation that creates a skewed distribution. The optimal choice would be to provide catastrophic coverage for all age groups in the population. To assure a normally distributed curve of health care costs, the program would have to be mandatory.

All other groups in the population should be provided with catastrophic coverage, including

1. The growing number of employees shifted from full-time to part-time employment by employers avoiding payments of fringe benefits
2. People who were covered while married through their spouse's group plan but who, after a specified time following a divorce, are unable to secure individual coverage because of a preexisting condition
3. Emancipated minors attending universities who rely totally on student health services because they cannot afford individual coverage
4. Persons who had group coverage when working for a corporation but left it to start a small business and cannot afford coverage or have a preexisting condition
5. Persons who do not qualify for Medicaid because they earn too much but who also cannot afford to purchase health insurance

Two problems need to be explored carefully if catastrophic coverage is provided across the board for all types of illness: (1) What monthly premium level would permit enrollment of the entire population? and (2) What would be the threshold level (in dollars) at which catastrophic coverage (including acute care, nursing home care, outpatient care, rehabilitation, and psychiatric services) would begin? The purpose of catastrophic coverage is to cap the amount of money an individual or his primary insurance company has to pay for medical care. The objective in establishing a threshold for catastrophic coverage is to set the base at the point at which only a small percentage of patients qualify. The higher the percentage of patients who reach the threshold, the higher the monthly premium must be set. It might be desirable in the early years of a national catastrophic program to give priority to the monthly premium cost and set the coverage accordingly, rather than the reverse. The primary question is, How much is an individual or employer willing to pay in order to have a known dollar level beyond which there are no additional costs for medical care? (A main advantage of a national catastrophic coverage program is that it would permit a free market to operate below the threshold level of catastrophic coverage. Commercial insurance, HMOs, Blue Cross, PPOs, Medicare, and Medicaid could still continue to compete and provide care.)

To keep the monthly premium modest, the focus has to be on what services can be provided at a low premium level. If the focus is allowed to shift to the comprehensiveness of care and broadened to cover other services such as nursing homes, prescription drugs, and other incidental health services, the monthly premium will rise significantly, with the risk that increasing portions of the population will not purchase the coverage. If the premium rate was held low and benefits gradually expanded to a wider range of services, the government might once again find itself paying for more health care than it can afford with its budgetary constraints.

The need for a reliable database in catastrophic coverage is of such importance that coverage should initially be limited to acute hospital care and the associated professional fees, until the utilization data are sufficiently refined to permit the development of a sound actuarial basis for determining premiums. No data exists for comparing the cost of care in nursing homes, rehabilitation programs, psychiatric institutions, and home health programs, and the cost of prescription drugs. No one really knows how much nursing home care might be used if available through catastrophic coverage. To include other elements of care without knowing their use rates would financially defeat the purpose of the program. Demonstration projects for these additional programs in the geographical areas where they would be implemented would be needed to develop a reliable database for actuarial purposes.

Use of a Monthly Deductible

For a national program to be successful, the monthly premium must meet two criteria: (1) it must be a modest dollar amount that is acceptable to all segments of the population, and (2) the method of payment must be easy. The best avenue to explore would be a standard paycheck deduction, such as that now taken by the Social Security Administration. The existing rules for collecting social security taxes could be applied to the collection of health care premiums from part-time and full-time employees, and like the social security tax, the health care premium could be mandatory for the total employed population. A formula that might be considered is the following:

(ANNUAL EMPLOYER AND EMPLOYEE
SOCIAL SECURITY CONTRIBUTIONS OF AN
INDIVIDUAL ÷ 12 MONTHS) × HEALTH SPENDING
AS A PERCENTAGE OF GDP

Two examples illustrate this method:

Example 1

1. The individual's maximum taxable income under Social Security is $57,600.
2. The combined employer/employee Social Security contribution at 15 percent is $8,640.
3. $8,640 divided by twelve months is $720.
4. $720 multiplied by the health spending percentage of the GDP (13.5 percent) is $97.20.
5. The person's monthly health care deductible is $97.20. Spending for the year is $1,166.40 (the maximum amount if used every month).

Example 2

1. An individual earns $20,000 per year.
2. The combined employer/employee Social Security contribution at 15 percent is $3,000.
3. $3,000 divided by twelve months is $250.
4. $250 multiplied by the health spending percentage of the GDP (13.5 percent) is $33.75.
5. The person's monthly health care deductible is $33.75. Spending for the year is $405 (the maximum amount if used every month).

Standardizing the deductible through the use of a formula assures fairness, but at the same time it provides a deductible that varies from year to year based on the combined Social Security contribution and fluctuations in the health care component of the GDP. The application of the deductible could be made either mandatory or optional for carriers, both government and private industry. If optional, each financing mechanism would be free to determine its own payment method. CHAMPUS and Medicare, for example, might elect to continue existing benefits unchanged, while Blue Cross, Blue Shield, and commercial carriers might elect to apply a deductible. Conversely, making the deductible mandatory would have the following advantages:

- It would create a level playing field for all participants.
- It would communicate a belief that a national policy is an important link between the health care system and economic consequences.
- The deductible corridor for carriers would be standardized.
- For disadvantaged patients, vouchers would not only serve to enroll an individual in a local plan at the basic benefits level, but would eliminate the requirement for a co-insurance feature.

Coverage should also be available to self-employed persons, as well as persons not employed but wishing to participate as individuals. In addition, local and state governments would be eligible to make contributions for Medicaid recipients (for whom Medicaid pays rates so low that hospitals and physicians do not want to take care of them) and would make these patients financially acceptable to health care providers. Thus, coverage would be available to the entire population.

Payment to Providers

Yet to be determined is the method of payment to hospital providers. Experience indicates that cost reimbursement is unsatisfactory as a method of payment. Equally unsatisfactory is the DRG method, because of the abuses that have been initiated by the HCFA. Though more cumbersome, a satisfactory solution might be a rate negotiated annually by HCFA (or its intermediaries) and individual hospitals. In some communities it might be desirable for hospitals to bid competitively for catastrophic patients. If so, hospitalized patients would be transferred to contract hospitals when catastrophic coverage commenced. In most instances, a transfer would be safe if a patient's condition were stable; the primary focus would be on the economics of medical care.

It is important, however, to provide care at the catastrophic level with as little disruption as possible in the continuum of patient care. It would be desirable to not require a patient to be transferred to another program or facility simply to satisfy the financing mechanism. Rather than transfer a patient, the provider could charge the federal catastrophic fund the same amount as the lowest rate it would charge a commercial carrier. Retrospective audits would make this approach relatively easy to monitor. It would have the advantage of not requiring the federal government to determine rates by geographic areas or based on rural/urban differences. If this approach proved effective, the rates would be set by marketplace conditions in each community. The federal government would simply take advantage of the lowest available rate. However, since contract rates are subject to change, the federal program would need to require that the individual catastrophic contract with a provider remain in place for one year before being subject to change.

Determining Minimum Benefits

Assuming that the federal government adopts a plan of mandatory health care coverage for all citizens, additional questions need to be answered:

1. How extensive should minimum benefits be?
2. How is a minimum benefit program to be audited to ensure that all citizens are participating?
3. What sources of funding can be used?

Determining the extent of minimum benefits is a difficult task when such benefits are determined based on the type of care provided. A wide variety of programs offering coverage are already in place, some sponsored by the federal government, others by for-profit and not-for-profit organizations, from the CHAMPUS program, Medicare, and Medicaid to Blue Cross/Blue Shield and commercial carriers. Why not permit all insuring sources to remain in place as long as they meet minimum standards of coverage? Existing benefits under each plan could be converted to dollars of coverage similar to indemnity coverages.

The issues involved in determining minimum benefits are quite different from the issues involved in determining whether to provide catastrophic coverage. The development of a catastrophic program fills a gap that is largely missing today. Little concern is necessary that it duplicates existing coverages, and a plan could be implemented with relative ease with minimum disruption to existing coverages.

Conclusions

The purpose of the national health care program proposed here would be to increase the public's trust in the medical care system, not to solve all of the fiscal issues. The program would provide maximum financial support to patients who face financial disaster from prolonged or expensive illness. It is designed to maintain a free-market operation, while at the same time providing a method for covering the uninsured.

To attempt to answer all of the country's health care needs with an all-encompassing elegant solution that standardizes what all people will receive would surely lead away from and not toward the desired result. The public will not support only one system. Therefore, an incremental, carefully thought-out public policy would seem to be a more desirable route to follow.

If a major restructuring of health care is to take place in the near future, with access to health care significantly increased but without commensurate funding, hospitals will need to develop a strategic view in order to avoid decreasing public trust as patients blame hospitals for problems created by government policy. Rather than waiting for legislative proposals to be introduced, hospitals and their representatives need to have a strong voice in shaping the future of the health care system. Such initiative is a responsibility that should not be left solely to hospital and physician associations, but should include the thoughtful input of those on the firing line (patients, employee benefits managers, and so on). Experienced judgment is needed to advocate the enactment of catastrophic coverage as a first step, rather than attempting to deal with all of the complex dimensions of health care at the same time. This proposed approach is a major step toward protecting the public from ruinous financial consequences of illness, while leaving other problems to be dealt with in the future when more information and statistics are available to guide sound decision making.

How does the public's trust in hospitals relate to the restructuring of the financing of health care? The public is of two minds. It gives hospitals high marks as institutions of healing, but it has serious misgivings about hospitals as economic entities, because of the financial perils that accompany illness. This dilemma is now a major concern on the public's agenda. Depending on decisions that are likely to be reached in the near future by the federal establishment, the public's regard for hospitals will increase or decrease substantially. A shift in public attitude will occur with any major change that Congress decides to enact. The public reaction to whatever is enacted will take place in two time frames. In the short run, if access to health care is made widely available and global budgeting adopted to assure "reasonable costs," there will be a great sense of public relief, and a new confidence in hospitals will develop. If, however, "reasonable costs" become too onerous for providers and result in long waiting times, poorer quality, and lagging technology, the long-term outlook will be a loss in public confidence. Conversely, if reasonable costs permit hospitals to maintain existing levels of service, a win-win situation will have been created and public confidence will return.

Chapter Four

Straws in the Wind or Where Is the Health Field Headed?

Richard L. Johnson

What major health care changes are likely over the next two decades? The role of Medicare and Medicaid programs will change. Managed care's future with capitation and its acceptance by the public will shift. Hospitals will have several different perspectives: on the development of systems, the need for beds, the role of affiliated systems, the for-profit hospital, the future of the freestanding hospital, and finally, cost shifting. Physician interaction with managed care and hospitals will change in the years ahead, and public attitudes toward health care will be different.

Modifications and adjustments to ongoing activities are not what is needed. Adding to or subtracting from what is ongoing in the operating organization is no longer a way of getting ready for the future. To avoid failure, a willingness to take substantial risk is now necessary. To believe that simply continuing to do what has been successful in the past will work in the future is to deny the realities of the current marketplace. Clinging to what was will not solve the problems now emerging. Self-criticism and self-questioning must now become the starting point for change. The challenge is not simply to do better; it is to reinvent; to develop new corporate structures and new relationships, and to find new opportunities; to become a totally different health care organization.

The Current State of Affairs

Hospitals and physicians are currently rushing headlong into managed care and capitation. Physicians are leaving solo practices, forming single-specialty and multispecialty group practices, being employed by hospitals and managed care plans, and developing various practice organizations, all in an effort to attain sufficient clout to deal with managed care. Hospitals are affiliating with health care systems, selling out to both for-profit and not-for-profit systems, and at the same time integrating with physicians into physician-hospital organizations (PHOs). The driving force behind all of these provider activities is that managed care is becoming so large and important in the financing of health care that providers also have to become large and important or no longer be a factor in the marketplace.

There is a perception among both hospital executives and physicians that capitation will become the primary payment mechanism. A comment frequently heard from chief executives of hospitals is that they are getting ready for capitation. In a March 1995 hospital survey conducted by one of the authors of this book at the TriBrook Group, a health care consulting firm founded by the author in 1972, 75 percent of the respondents indicated that they believe capitation will become the major source of hospital revenues. Both freestanding hospitals and solo-practice physicians have become concerned that the future holds increasing financial problems, and possibly their elimination as providers. The belief that survival depends on becoming increasingly larger gained considerable strength following the demise of the Clinton administration's proposal for a national health system. When health care reform died in Congress in 1994, the events that followed—the mergers and consolidations of hospitals, the formation of more systems and alliances, the rapid increase in business coalitions, PHOs, POs, and IPAs—seemed to be an unleashing of the entrepreneurial and competitive forces that are now at large.

The interest in managed care has been fueled by a Congressional belief that under this form of payment patients will continue to receive high quality care while the monthly premium levels off. Congressional leaders have indicated that they believe they can reduce projected Medicare payments by $270 billion over the next seven years and, for good measure, that an additional $183 billion can be eliminated from projected Medicaid spending as Congress moves to balance the federal budget. Between what Congress is doing now and the public's expectations about what managed care can accomplish is a widespread belief that the solution to the health care "crisis" may be at hand. Thoughtful physicians and hospital executives share the same expectations as the public, though they may be somewhat more pessimistic. Despite these expectations and hopes for the future, there are enough "straws in the wind" to raise considerable doubt about what may come to pass. A far different reality may take place.

Unanticipated shifts will take place as the public, providers, and government officials come to appreciate that their understandings of the trends at work are incomplete and, as problems arise, unexpected. A number of these straws in the wind have already become apparent, and will become more important in the days ahead. As they gain momentum as independent problems, they will eventually be viewed as facets of a larger problem and will lead to a shift away from the trends that now seem to be inevitable. As new trends develop, they will bump against each other and eventually set a new direction for the health care field. Each of the five major players—the government, managed care organizations, hospitals, physicians, and the public—will have to deal separately with its own set of problems, and then with how it is impacted by the other four players. The following sections will examine the problems associated with each of the players separately, and then look at how they are interrelated.

The Government

With the change in party leadership in both the House of Representatives and the Senate in late 1994, concerns about the growing federal deficit suddenly found new support. Proposals to reduce the size of the national debt by downsizing government have focused attention on the Medicare and Medicaid programs. The congressional time frame proposes to achieve these reductions over seven years by limiting increases to five percent per year. However, in the proposed seven-year period (1995 to 2002), the sixty-five-plus age group will increase by 2,322,000 persons.[1] The result for hospitals will be an increased shortfall in revenue. Even though the total dollars in the Medicare program will increase each year (10 percent of Medicare funds are spent for disabled persons, 88 percent for enrollees (those sixty-five and older), and 2 percent for administrative costs of the program), the cost to hospitals for providing services to Medicare patients will also increase, at a rate of 10.2 percent per year, and at the same time the number of persons enrolled in Medicare will also increase. Medicare patients currently account for 44 percent of all of the days of care provided in acute care hospitals. Based on averages determined from all health maintenance organization (HMO) data,[2] approximately 1,700 hospital days are used annually per one thousand Medicare members. The HMO averages indicate that expenditures per HMO enrollee are close to $700 annually, of which physicians receive 57 percent and hospitals receive 43 percent.

The Congressional Budget Office (CBO) released a report in August 1995, "The Economic and Budget Outlook, Fiscal Years 1996–2000." The report projects anticipated Medicare expenditures that can be compared to Congressional planning (see Table 4.1). In the years 2001 and 2002, a savings of $95 billion is anticipated. Table 4.2 shows the impact of this projection on the average Medicare expenditure per enrollee as intended by Congress.

Table 4.3 relates the data for 1995 to the CBO and congressional projections for 2000. Using the CBO projection, the payment per day from Medicare would rise $656 during the five-year period, but using the congressional goal, the increase would be $262 per day. If hospitals are able to limit their increase per year to 5 percent (assuming that this is the rate of inflation), the amount received from Medicare will be $1,488 or $60 per day, a differential in five years of 4 percent.

Because Medicare patient days are such a substantial source of hospital revenues, hospitals cannot afford to eliminate Medicare admissions; but if they exceed cost increases of more than 5 percent per year, some hospitals may be forced out of business. If enough hospitals are unable to contain their costs, financial leverage ultimately will shift from the buyer to the provider. If this occurs, the federal programs may have to reconsider their payment levels or refocus the program.

Table 4.1. Projected Expenditures for Medicare.

Year	CBO Projections	Percentage Increase	Congressional Intent	Difference
1994 Actual	$160B	—	$160B	—
1995 Projected	176B	10.1 percent	176B	—
1996 Projected	196B	11.2	185B	$9B
1997 Projected	217B	9.7	194B	23B
1998 Projected	238B	8.9	204B	34B
1999 Projected	262B	9.2	214B	48B
2000 Projected	286B	8.4	225B	61B
				$175B

Source: U.S. Congress, Congressional Budget Office. *The Economic and Budget Outlook: Fiscal Years 1996–2000.* Washington, D.C.: Congressional Budget Office, 1995.

Table 4.2. Projected Expenditure per Enrollee.

Year	Number of Enrollees	CBO Projections	Congressional Intent	Expenditure per Enrollee per Year
1995	33.6M	$176B	—	$5,238
2000	35.0	286B	—	$8,171
2000	35.0	—	$225B	$6,428

Managed Care

In July 1994, approximately 43.4 million persons, or 16.7 percent of the 260 million people in the United States, were enrolled in traditional HMOs. Such enrollment is expected to rise to between 58.5 and 68 million by mid 1997,[3] which will represent between 21 and 25 percent of the population. Some advocates of managed care are predicting enrollments of 48 percent out of a population of 276 million in the year 2000, or 132.5 million people covered by managed care plans. A study conducted by Lewin VHI and Associates[4] reported that the original projections of 48 percent would,

Table 4.3. Projected Funding Available to Hospitals from Medicare.

	Actual 1995	CBO 2000	Congress 2000
Medicare expenditures	$176B	$286B	$225B
Percentage of funds for hospitals and physicians	×.88	×.88	×.88
Total available for hospitals and physicians	$155B	$252B	$198B
Percentage for hospitals	×.43	×.43	×.43
Total funding for hospitals	$66.6B	$108.4B	$85.0B
Enrollees	33.6M	35.0M	35.0M
Average patient days per 1,000 patients	×1,700	×1,700	×1,700
Annual patient days	57.12M	59.5M	59.5M
Hospital revenue per day	$1,166	$1,822	$1,428

Source: Marion Merrell Dow. *Managed Care Digest, Update Edition 1994.* Kansas City, Mo.: Marion Merrell Dow, 1994, p. 4. Used with permission of Marion Merrell Dow and SMG Marketing Group.

as a result of willing provider laws, be held to 31 percent, or 85.6 million people enrolled in plans by the year 2000. Managed care plans would thus need to enroll an additional 16 to 27 million persons by the turn of the century. To achieve the more optimistic increase of 48 percent, enrollments in that same period would need to increase by 63.5 to 74.5 million over and above the Interstudy projections of 58.5 to 68 million, and the total number of enrolled would need to be between 106.9 and 117.9 million people. Such growth rates of 2.5 to 2.7 times current levels seem wildly off the mark and suggest overly enthusiastic support for managed care.

Interstudy reported that in 1994 the Medicare population enrolled in managed care was 6.1 percent of 31 million Medicare recipients aged sixty-five and older.[5] By 2000, 35 million Americans will be sixty-five and older, and if 6.1 percent are enrolled in managed care, 2.1 million elders will be covered. It seems reasonable to believe that by the year 2000, 30 percent of the under-sixty-five population may be enrolled in managed care, which would amount to 72 million persons, and if the sixty-five-and-older cohort is included, a total of about 74 million people will be enrolled, a difference of 32.9 to 43.9 million persons fewer than the 48 percent predicted by advocates of managed care (see Figure 4.1).

It has been suggested in congressional circles that managed care should be mandated for Medicare enrollees, but others in Congress have indicated that they feel individuals should be allowed to make this decision themselves. Congressional comments to the press have indicated that there is substantial resistance to the idea of forced participation, and it is unlikely that it will be required.

It is anticipated that capitation will eventually be the preferred method of payment for managed care. Currently, the use of capitation as a method of paying for hospital services and for care by specialists has not grown significantly and is still a minor form of payment, as shown in Tables 4.4 and 4.5. However, as shown in Table 4.6, capitation is the primary method of payment for primary care.

Capitation is a system in which the subscriber pays a monthly premium to the managed care plan, which in turn contracts with physicians and hospitals to provide all needed services for a fixed

Figure 4.1. Projected HMO Enrollments.

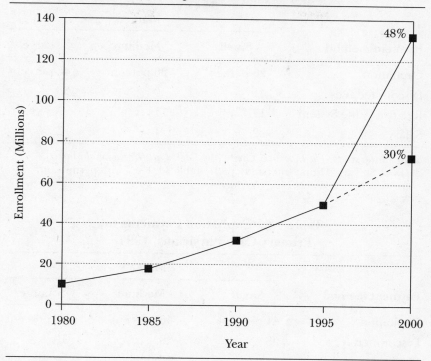

Source: Interstudy. *The Interstudy Competitive Edge, Part III: Regional Market Analysis.* St. Paul, Minn.: Interstudy, p. 31, Table 14. Used with permission.

Table 4.4. Capitation Payments to Hospitals, 1994.

Payment method	Markets		
	Small	**Medium**	**Large**
Capitation	8 percent	11 percent	12 percent
Per diem	40	34	36
DRG	15	15	18
Discounted fee	22	17	15

Source: Interstudy. *The Interstudy Competitive Edge, Part III: Regional Market Analysis.* St. Paul, Minn.: Interstudy, p. 31, Table 14. Used with permission.

Table 4.5. Capitation Payments to Specialists, 1994.

Payment method	Markets		
	Small	Medium	Large
Capitation	26 percent	26 percent	46 percent
Discounted fees	41	40	33
Relative Value System	17	11	5
Salary	2	1	2

Source: Interstudy. *The Interstudy Competitive Edge, Part III: Regional Market Analysis.* St. Paul, Minn.: Interstudy, p. 31, Table 14. Used with permission.

Table 4.6. Capitation Payments to Primary-Care Physicians, 1994.

Payment method	Markets		
	Small	Medium	Large
Capitation	41 percent	46 percent	63 percent
Discounted fees	23	23	19
RVS	14	7	2
Salary	10	4	3

Source: Interstudy. *The Interstudy Competitive Edge, Part III: Regional Market Analysis.* St. Paul, Minn.: Interstudy, p. 31, Table 14. Used with permission.

amount of money per month. The managed care plan is in an enviable position. It collects the monthly premiums, takes out its expenses and profits, and then passes on the remaining dollars to the providers. In communities in which there are far too many empty hospital beds, capitation forces hospitals to bid for managed care contracts based on marginal costs (the direct cost of adding the last day of patient care) rather than on average costs (direct and indirect expenses totaled and divided by the number of adjusted patient days). As long as capitation remains a small percentage of hospital revenue, hospitals can afford to bid based on marginal cost. However, if capitation becomes a major source of revenue, hospitals will have to forego bidding on this basis, and over time they will be unable to continue to cost shift to make up for lost revenue. Coupling managed care capitation with the proposed limitations on Medicare revenues within the next few years would force hospitals to apply average costs when bidding for contracts. Marginal costs would no longer be feasible. Managed care plans would then be faced with higher and higher payments to those hospitals that remained open, once the supply and the demand for acute beds was back in balance. When that time arrives, it will be necessary to search for alternatives to managed care. When hospitals recognize that they must apply average cost in bidding, they will require managed care plans to guarantee an annual number of days of care so that they are assured of revenues at a level that permits them to effectively budget their resources.

This shift in leverage from managed care plans to providers will not take place until the supply of staffed beds is balanced with the need for beds. In the meantime, the trade journals and the public media will be reporting on the continued growth of managed care plans. While growth in enrollment will be accelerating, the number of plans will be decreasing as larger and better-financed plans buy up their competition. The Twin Cities of Minnesota—where the number of plans has steadily decreased over the past ten years and is now at three—provide a good example of what will occur among managed care plans as they mature in various markets.

Of the 547 HMOs currently in operation,[6] 69 percent (380) are for-profit. This segment will become larger as Blue Cross creates for-profit managed care plans and as larger HMOs absorb smaller plans. In the competitive marketplace of managed care, consolidations occur when plans have large reserves and use them to obtain additional markets. In addition, many plans will purchase physician practices but not hospitals. Ownership of managed care plans will enable HMOs to exert control over which hospitals are used for their subscribers.

Eventually, managed care will run its course, be recognized for its limitations, and probably top out with an enrollment of around 35 percent of the population. This may take place at about the beginning of the next century, as public dissatisfaction reaches the point where alternatives will be sought. To some degree, the dissatisfaction will be brought on by the way managed care plans measure their success. The trade journals regularly report patient days per one thousand managed-care enrollees for two groups: those under sixty-five years old and those sixty-five and older. The numbers are routinely compared by plan executives. Comparative data on utilization rates are used to evaluate plan efficiency, with the goal of achieving lower and lower utilization. If a competing plan has, for example, a ten percent lower utilization, the goal becomes to beat the competition with a better score. The appropriateness and timing of the care provided are less important considerations. Because appropriateness and timing are difficult to measure, they have been a lower priority for managed care executives. This pattern will continue until the public, in substantial numbers, reaches the point where they sue managed care plans and their physicians for not providing adequate care. When that point is reached, the public will seek alternatives to managed care, and many will turn to hospital systems.

Hospitals

For the next several years, the hospital field is likely to be on a for-profit kick, which will have two components: the for-profit health care chains will remain for-profit, and the nonprofit affiliated health care systems will become for-profit. Eventually, both components will be integrated systems.

Freestanding and Affiliated Nonprofit Hospitals

The nonprofit affiliated systems and freestanding nonprofit hospitals of today will likely become for-profit organizations. This will occur for three reasons: (1) affiliations are weak organizations; (2) equity funds are needed to accomplish the desired results; and (3) when joining systems, physicians will push for for-profit status as a way of offsetting declining patient revenue as managed care plans restrict payments to physicians.

As the economic era of health care emerges, the day of the freestanding hospital draws to a close. Concerned with attracting managed care contracts, hospitals have come to appreciate that consolidations and mergers are necessary if they are to remain competitive. Their multiple governing boards are being collapsed into one central board for important decision making. Independent hospitals and solo physician practices are turning into integrated systems with multiple sites. Where PHOs are being created, they are most often for-profit entities. Increasingly, the PHO or its equivalent that combines physicians and hospitals will become the dominant provider as it obtains managed care contracts. The ability to capture a revenue stream, rather than the ability to generate revenues to be put back into brick and mortar, will become of primary importance. The economic reality being faced by physicians and hospitals is that the difference between winners and losers will be the ability to attract managed care contracts.

Even though nearly two-thirds of primary care physicians now receive capitation in large markets and nearly half of specialists in the same markets are paid by capitation, only 12 percent of hospitals are paid by this mechanism (see Tables 4.4, 4.5, and 4.6). As capitation becomes less popular with the public, physician and hospital dislike of this method of payment will also increase until they turn away from it. However, by that time hospitals and health care systems will have gained enough understanding of managed care that they will approach employers with offers to deal directly with them and cut out the carriers, thereby eliminating the 15 to 20 percent that the carriers skim off the top of premium payments.

The combined nonprofit and for-profit hospital systems now control 37.5 percent of the 880,000 staffed hospital beds in the United States. Of the 329,608 system beds, the for-profit systems control 36 percent, which represents 13.5 percent of all beds. It should be recognized that there are significant differences between for-profit and nonprofit ownership. In the for-profit sector, the corporate office clearly controls the financial operations, but in nonprofit affiliations only very limited authority is granted to the central organization. Assets and liabilities are not comingled, but the affiliated hospitals rely on voluntary agreements aimed at successfully bidding for managed care contracts.

The ability of affiliations to survive in the face of the kind of financial pressure that can be brought to bear by managed care plans is questionable. There is a notable reluctance among nonprofit hospitals to give up their autonomy. By only affiliating, rather than giving up ownership, they retain control, but this approach pits a loose, weak organizational structure against centrally controlled managed care plans when negotiating contracts. In an economic climate in which hospitals have too many surplus beds and lower-than-desirable occupancy rates, it is likely that managed care plans will dominate the negotiating activities in dealing with hospitals.

The strategy of managed care plans depends on getting as low a price as possible, so they often attempt to break up affiliations by offering larger volumes of patients to selected units of the affiliation in return for a more favorable price. Once an affiliation agreement has been breached, it may be difficult for the affiliated system to avoid breaking up.

In the future, the hospital may well remain nonprofit, but the central activities of the health care delivery system will of necessity have to become for-profit. Still, the influence of the nonprofit hospital may be sufficiently strong that the integrated delivery system will behave on the basis of the traditional nonprofit values rather than according to the values of the for-profit systems now on the health care scene. If individual unit governing boards are left in place, they will have only restricted authority, such as being limited to medical credentialing and oversight of quality of care but lacking the authority to commit funds.

Because of the difficulty of changing from an affiliated structure to a central controlling structure, it appears that affiliations are a passing phenomenon of the health care field. The result of their passing could be a nonprofit, centrally controlled system, but this is unlikely. Because of the speed with which integrated delivery systems are developing, those that are successful will recognize that acquiring additional hospitals and other health-related activities requires spending a great deal of money in a relatively short period of time. To do so requires using equity dollars. Relying on long-term debt and cash reserves will not be sufficient; investors will be needed, requiring a for-profit corporate structure.

For-Profit Health Care Systems

To build health care systems that include multiple activities at multiple sites and that include physician services, those systems with such a vision will become for-profit and be the major force in health care. Though the hospital itself may remain nonprofit, its role will no longer be central. It will be replaced by the for-profit system that has been built in a relatively short number of years using equity money to put all of the pieces in place. The driving force behind this development will be physicians and health care executives, not the community-minded hospital trustee.

One of the major reasons that for-profit health care systems are growing rapidly is their willingness to purchase nonprofit and public hospitals at a price that is often 50 percent higher than bids from nonprofit competitors. This approach is not being reported in health care journals, but it is a reality encountered by a nonprofit hospital when preparing a bid to buy another freestanding hospital that has been put up for sale in a nearby service area, and it is likely to continue until most hospitals have been absorbed into systems. Then the situation will change, but until then, the for-profit chains will continue to bid higher prices for hospital facilities.

For-profit chains march to a different drumbeat than nonprofit chains. Their decisions are made with an eye on Wall Street, not Main Street. By paying higher prices, they are able to put new acquisitions on their balance sheets at inflated prices, which in turn increases the value per share of stock and is therefore attractive to investors. It also increases the value of the portfolios of the executives who own large blocks of their own stock. The payment of higher prices by for-profit chains will continue until the well of available hospitals begins to dry up, at which point for-profit chain executives will realize that the future of their companies will be determined by the profit margin from operations and not by a rise in stock prices. At that point consideration will be given to the sale of the for-profit hospital corporation. As insiders, executives must report sales of their stock to the Securities Exchange Commission, which will make the sale public information. Because of such disclosure laws, executives will hold the bulk of their shares until the company is sold.

The premiums that for-profit chains have paid to purchase hospitals work well as long as the marketplace for buying hospitals exists. Continuing increases in capital assets is an inducement to investors to buy shares. When a price per share of stock steadily rises, it looks like a sound investment. However, when the number of hospitals for sale dries up or surplus beds remain empty, the investor's attention shifts from the rising price per share to paying attention to the return on the investment (ROI). Making an adequate ROI will be more difficult in coming years because of the restraints being placed on Medicare and Medicaid payments by the federal government and because of the ability of managed care plans to reduce outlays to providers because of their growing share of the marketplace. The result is predictable. Several years from now, stock prices of for-profit chains will decline substantially over a short period, and there may well be a fire sale of these hospitals as a result of the inflated prices that were paid in putting the system together. Paying inflated prices to purchase hospitals works to the advantage of for-profit systems for now, but it is not beyond reason to believe that when these companies are confronted with decreasing revenues and a decline in stock prices, there will be an economic collapse among for-profit systems.

Utilization

Table 4.7 provides data on the steady decline in the use of hospital beds since 1983. The trends forecast for the year 2000 are the results of the likely changes. If no additional beds are added to hospital systems in the next five years, by the year 2000 system beds would constitute 40 percent of all staffed beds (329,608 of 821,250), due to the continued decline in staffed beds. If revenues to hospitals are restricted, the occupancy of staffed beds is likely to hold at 65 percent in order to obtain a reasonable degree of efficiency. The result in the year 2000 would be 750,000 beds in operation, or 44 percent of all beds in hospital systems with no net additions.[7]

Recognizing that hospital systems will continue to grow and expand, it is easy to conceive that 80 percent of all staffed beds will be in systems by the year 2000, so that 600,000 beds out of 750,000 beds will be included. To achieve this result, 54,078 beds in freestanding hospitals would need to be added to system beds in each of the next five years. To acquire these beds at $100,000 per bed would require systems to pay $5.4 billion per year for the next five years, an amount that is doable.

One of the keys to the future of health care lies in determining the utilization rates that will be acceptable to the public, employers, and federal programs in the year 2000. Table 4.8 shows the number of patient days of care in hospitals that will be needed

Table 4.7. Decline in Bed Usage.

Year	Staffed Beds	Patient Days	Average Occupancy	U.S. Population	Patient Days/1,000
1983	1,021,000	273,536,000	73.4 percent	233.3M	1,172
1988	949,000	226,882,170	63.5	244.5M	928
1993	921,000	216,445,000	64.4	257.9M	839
1995	880,000	206,020,000**	64.2	263.4M	782
Difference	−141,000	−67,516,000	−9.2 percent	+30.1M	−390
2000	821,250	177,900,000	59.3 percent	276.2M*	644
65 and older		78,300,000		35.3M*	2167
Under 65		99,600,000		240.9M*	421

* Projection is Middle series.

** Estimate by author.

Source: U.S. Bureau of the Census, *Statistical Abstract of the United States: 1994* (114th ed.). Washington, D.C.: Department of Commerce, 1994, Tables 15 and 16; American Hospital Association. *Hospital Statistics: 1994.* Chicago, Ill.: American Hospital Association, 1994, Table 1.

Table 4.8. Projected Patient Days of Care in 2000.

	2000 Population	Utilization Rate	Patient Days
Under 65 HMO (30 percent)	72.3M	296.8	21.5M
Over 65 HMO (6.1 percent)	2.1	1,697	3.6
Under 65	168.6	421	70.9
Over 65	33.2	2,167	71.9
Total	276.2M		167.9M

Source: Marion Merrell Dow. *Managed Care Digest, HMO Edition, 1994.* Kansas City, Mo.: Marion Merrell Dow, 1994, pp. 24, 25. Used with permission of Marion Merrell Dow and SMG Marketing Group.

if 30 percent of the population under age sixty are enrolled in HMOs and 6.1 percent of the Medicare group are also enrolled. It is reasonable to conclude that by the year 2000 the impact of HMO coverage of 30 percent will reduce patient days by an additional 10 million and decrease utilization to 608 days per 1,000 population. This would result in an overall occupancy rate of 61.3 percent based on 750,000 beds in service. Given a need to maintain a more efficient operation because of shortfalls in revenue, the number of staffed beds in 2000 possibly could decrease to 575,000 in order to maintain an 80 percent occupancy rate. This would be a decrease of 305,000 beds, which seems unlikely in a five-year period.

Physicians

With the development of managed care has come the concept of the *gatekeeper,* a primary care physician who determines when a patient needs to be seen by a specialist. The gatekeeper is part of an economic model, not a medical model, in which primary care physicians are encouraged to provide as much of the care as possible and to limit referrals to specialists.

The use of capitation has led to a number of difficulties for physicians. Specialists recognize that their dependence on primary care physicians has increased, because fewer specialists are needed. With the reduced volume of referrals, competition among specialists for patients increases. This has led to the development in some states of "willing provider" laws, whereby physicians cannot be excluded from contracting with a managed care plan as long as they meet the criteria for participation. The number of such laws may increase, in spite of managed care opposition and because of public opinion supporting patients' free choice of physicians.

Many physicians are not fond of managed care because it forces them to consider economics as well as medical needs, which may make them feel compromised in deciding on a course of treatment for a patient. This conflict also creates a barrier between primary care physicians and specialists. Primary care physicians have clinical breadth, while specialists have clinical depth. The choice is between an economic model and a medical model. A medical model gives precedence to accuracy, timeliness of clinical decisions, and effectiveness of treatment protocols, based on in-depth knowledge of what is needed. Rather than seeking economic models that retain and utilize these skills, managed care tends, in the interest of cost control, to substitute economic concerns for medical concerns. Ultimately, this attitude will become a public issue, as patients file suits against primary care physicians and managed care plans on the grounds that a properly trained physician would have had a better result. As capitation becomes increasingly unpopular with the public, frustrated patients and awards for damages for not providing appropriate medical care will bring about modifications in the capitation system.

The Public

The rise of managed care and the restrictions it places on the use of health care resources have been the result of yearly escalations in monthly premium costs that exceeded the rate of inflation. These escalations led representatives of the public to seek ways to moderate such increases by adopting mechanisms that intruded on the doctor-patient relationship. Both employers and the federal government felt the need to adopt cost-control measures and turned away from unregulated fee-for-service payments to physicians and hospitals. With increasing frequency, the managed care model appeared to offer a solution. As prepayment organizations recognized the shift that was taking place, they began to develop alternatives to their traditional lines of business in response to the demands for change. What was happening in California and the Twin Cities—the two areas with the highest concentrations of population in managed care plans—became the model.

Hospitals and physicians recognized that the old ways of doing business were rapidly being outdated and that they needed to be responsive to what was happening. Traditional resistance to change by providers was replaced with a fear that if changes were not made the providers would soon be out of business. The fear that gripped them turned into panic to get on board as they saw the necessity to adjust to the new demands as quickly as possible. This panic led to a belief among providers that the public unquestioningly supported managed care and its offspring, capitation. Providers rushed to develop responses that they believed would enable them to deal on a level playing field with managed care plans. To date, little attention is being paid to the question, What does the public really demand of its health care system and how best can these demands be met?

Careful attention to and close examination of the trends at work leads to the impression that the future of health care is likely to be quite different from what is now envisioned. Capitation has two built-in problems that the public will gradually recognize as unacceptable: the lack of free choice of a physician and the inability to self-refer to a specialist. Employers are reluctant to force employees to select a physician from a list supplied by a managed care plan. If premiums increase no faster than the rate of inflation, employers may not require capitation in their negotiations for a contract with a carrier. These concerns are now leading to the rapid expansion of point-of-service plans, even though they require a modest payment by the patient.

The use of physician gatekeepers will ultimately lead to patient dissatisfaction with the requirement of having to see a primary care physician in order to access the services of a specialist, particularly when the patient is aware of the type of specialty services needed. To the extent that patients become aware that primary care physicians may benefit financially by not referring to specialists, patients will become increasingly dissatisfied with this limitation.

As patients learn more about managed care, they will come to understand that managed care executives are interested primarily in attaining the lowest possible utilization rates relative to the results obtained by their competition throughout the country. Both employers and patients will eventually appreciate that the driving force of a managed care plan is not to achieve the most appropriate use of hospital and specialist services, but rather to use as few services as possible. With hospitals, primary care physicians, and specialists at full risk, the providers are at the mercy of the managed care plans. The public will be unaware that the cause of their dissatisfaction will be due to the managed care plans' methods of operation. When providers recognize that they are being blamed by the public for not meeting the public's expectations for care, the providers themselves will take steps to redress the situation. By the time this occurs, health care will be dominated by integrated health care delivery systems, which will opt to develop a strategy that eliminates the managed care plans. These systems will approach employers and business coalitions themselves, offering to deal directly with them. The arguments they will use with employers is that they can provide better service and more responsiveness to patient needs, more economically. They will point out to the purchasers of health care coverage that the 15 to 20 percent profits of managed care plans can be reduced substantially by dealing directly with the providers.

This form of provider activity is still a long way off. Managed care has not yet run its full course and become a mature industry. As long as the economic results are favorable and utilizations are not tightened to the point where negative public reactions become widespread, the present trends will continue. It may well be a decade before provider organizations decide to move aggressively to take business away from managed care plans. This action will take place when the public asserts its desire for quality, access, and availability, and when they are satisfied that the costs of care are controlled sufficiently that cost is no longer the major factor.

Conclusions

Even though all five of the components described in this chapter have problems within themselves, they are also interrelated and have spin-off effects that will force each component to take the others into account. Because many of the trends now occurring in each of the components have not yet become full-blown, there will be a delay before they interact in a serious way with the others. However, the straws in the wind are now sufficiently clear as to enable some insights into what is likely to take place.

Short-Term Trends

Over the next few years, the dominance of economic factors will increase. Managed care and capitation will continue to be highly regarded by employers and government as the means of controlling the costs of health care. Hospitals will continue to join systems, either for-profit or nonprofit, or they will affiliate with other hospitals to aggregate their size in order to compete as equals with managed care. At the same time, they will develop PHOs, and management service organizations to integrate with the physician component. Within the next several years, most hospitals will be in systems and the rush to participate will be over. Likewise, solo physician practice will become history, and physicians will either be members of group practices or employed on salary by health care organizations. Contracts for provider services will control the relationships between those who pay for health care and those who provide it. Competition will intensify as these large organizations vie for market share.

While these trends among providers and the managed care plans are maturing, there will be a growing dissatisfaction among the public with regard to health care. Dissatisfaction will occur in several ways. The public will come to realize that capitation is an economic model and not a medical model, and that it leads to enormous profits for managed care companies. This realization will lead employers to seek alternatives, and when they are approached by integrated health care delivery systems wanting to deal with them directly, employers will in many cases terminate their managed care contracts. Employers will be willing to make this change because of the number of complaints they will be hearing from employees who have tales about being forced by contract terms to deal with primary care physicians when they have believed they should be treated by a specialist. Increasingly, as the public becomes disturbed with capitation, enrollment in these plans will slow down and may well top out at 35 percent of the population, which may create a climate favorable to integrated delivery systems stepping into a direct role with employers and groups.

The Long-Term Outlook

Pressure to reform the health care system will be eased by several factors. From a clinical perspective, ambulatory services will continue to develop, which will continue to decrease the need for acute care beds. At the same time, displeasure with the results of managed care will lead the public to find alternatives, which may include a modified return to fee-for-service and greater satisfaction with the care received from physicians, enhanced by a much closer working relationship between provider organizations and business coalitions. The predominance of health care systems will lead to the integration of many health care activities so that rather than have to deal with a fractionated health care system, the public will be able to access a "seamless" approach to their wide-ranging needs. In addition, the integrated delivery system will have incorporated a community health care information system (CHINS) that will give the public increased confidence when they need to use the health care network. By the time this system is in full swing, affiliated systems will have disappeared, and the number of hospitals and acute beds will have shrunk to an amount that balances need and supply.

The affiliated systems will have recognized that in a highly-competitive marketplace the ability to deal effectively with aggressive managed care plans is beyond the capability of the weak organizational structure of affiliations, and they will have been replaced with centrally controlled integrated delivery systems. As these systems mature and discover that full-risk capitation works only to the benefit of managed care plans, they will decide that they should enter into direct competition with these plans by dealing directly with employers and groups for their health care business. The need to engage in competition with managed care plans will come about as integrated delivery systems determine that they cannot continue to bid for contracts or accept Medicare payments that can only be obtained by resorting to marginal cost pricing. If they are to survive and prosper, they must use average costs.

What is evident, however, is that capitation will fall short of public expectations, and domination of the health care scene by large, integrated health care delivery systems may turn out to be the wave of the future. If this takes place, the antitrust laws will become a major factor in health care as a way of ensuring competition between the very large organizations that will dominate major markets. There is a feeling among hospital executives that antitrust laws are inappropriate in health care because the unnecessary duplication of expensive programs and services could be avoided to a great extent if hospitals were exempted from these regulations. This attitude will undergo a change after consolidations lead to a small number of health care delivery systems in a community. Those who pay for care will appreciate that no one system is permitted to dominate a local market. When only a limited number of survivors are present, antitrust laws will be viewed as necessary to protect the public's interest. In small towns and cities there may be only one survivor, but it will most likely be a unit of a system in the region and will be seen by the public as a health care resource that would otherwise not be available.

By the time the need has arisen to be supportive of antitrust laws, the supply of beds will not be back in balance with the need for beds, but the aggregate size of individual integrated systems will be large enough that the leverage needed to effectively negotiate revised upward payments from Medicare will be available. This leverage may in turn lead to congressional action to revamp the Medicare payment system. The willingness of the federal government to make such changes will have been influenced by the breakup of the for-profit delivery systems that were dependent upon continued expansion as the means of maintaining the interest of investors in buying their shares of stock. As these for-profit systems encounter financial difficulties and sell off pieces of the corporation, public opinion will shift away from the economic model back to the medical model. Whether this sets the stage for a national health system or leads in other directions will not be known for another decade or two.

Notes

1. U.S. Bureau of the Census. *Statistical Abstract of the United States: 1994* (114th ed.). Washington D.C.: Department of Commerce, Table 16, "Resident Population Projections, by Age and Sex: 1993 to 2050, Middle Series."

2. Marion Merrell Dow. *Managed Care Digest, Update Edition 1994.* Kansas City, Mo: Marion Merrell Dow, 1994.

3. Interstudy. *The Interstudy Competitive Edge, Part II: Industry Report.* St. Paul, Minn.: Interstudy, 1995, p. 7.

4. Lewin VHI and Associates. *The Wall Street Journal,* Dec. 18, 1995.

5. Interstudy. *The Interstudy Competitive Edge, Part III: Regional Market Analysis.* St. Paul, Minn.: Interstudy, 1995, p. 31, Table 14.

6. Marion Merrell Dow. *Managed Care Digest, HMO Edition 1994.* Kansas City, Mo.: Marion Merrell Dow, 1994.

7. American Hospital Association. *Hospital Statistics: 1994/95.* Chicago, Ill.: American Hospital Association, 1994, Table 1.

Chapter Five

Health Care Ethics in an Economic Era

Everett A. Johnson

When reading a hospital journal these days, one is likely to find an article describing how to develop a tighter relationship between a hospital and physicians that benefits both parties. Toward the end of these articles, there are usually one or two sentences that say, in effect, "by the way, be careful about the ethics involved."

Ethical standards are manifestations of moral principles that serve as day-to-day guides for determining personal and corporate behavior. In the past, to maintain public support the tradition and ethics of medical care placed the welfare and interests of patients foremost, and the interests of hospitals and physicians were seen as secondary. The public's expectation of ethical behavior in medical care defined the conduct of both the medical profession and the hospital organization, which delivered medical care as an expression of the moral standards of society. As long as the financing of medical care was essentially unlimited for both patients and providers, it was easy to maintain the existing ethical medical standard. However, a major shakeup in Medicare payments occurred in the mid 1980s, and both hospitals and physicians began seriously to seek out new ways to protect existing revenue levels and to develop new revenue sources. The result has been an expansion of business relationships between hospitals and physicians that has focused on economic incentives and bypassed traditional medical ethics. As competition for and regulatory pressures on medical services have increased, new public concerns have sporadically arisen about the ethical behavior toward patients of hospitals and physicians investing in joint ventures and other business and insurance arrangements.

As the public has become aware that some hospitals pay physicians for admitting patients to their facility or make nonrepayable loans to physicians, confidence in the integrity of hospitals and physicians has been lessened or lost.[1] When the public learns about joint ventures sponsored by hospitals and physicians that have large financial returns on limited investments, such as imaging centers, ambulatory surgery facilities, urgent care entities, home health care programs, and home intravenous services, public confidence is further reduced. Numerous examples of both excessive charges and overutilization of diagnostic laboratories have been reported.[2] For instance, a 1983 Michigan Blue Cross study reported that fees for laboratories owned by referring physicians were almost double the fees of other laboratories.

Less often recognized and discussed, but still open to questions about conflicts of interest, are investments by hospitals and physicians in jointly or separately sponsored health maintenance organizations (HMOs) and preferred provider organization (PPOs). Withholding a percentage of a physician's fee is customary practice for HMOs and PPOs. Physicians sponsored by an insurance carrier theoretically have an incentive to be judicious in their use of time and procedures. When a hospital and physicians jointly sponsor an HMO or PPO, it is assumed that they will be more motivated to practice conservative medical care than when sponsored by an insurance carrier, because their participation in profits will be more immediate and powerful; the assumption is that they will be more likely to encourage significant underutilization of medical care in order to reduce expenses. However, both medically sponsored HMOs and PPOs and carrier-sponsored programs have experienced financial collapse. These financial failures do not mean that the incentives are weak, but that physicians are more concerned about the health of patients than about the financial health of the organization. Physicians are trained to consider all of the diagnostic and treatment possibilities for a patient, so the economics of medical care becomes a secondary consideration.

Nevertheless, even though physicians' concerns are primarily clinical, the development of managed care programs and criteria may override physician decisions and compromise a patient's welfare. Fee-for-service medical practices allow physicians discretionary judgment, which provides a strong incentive for treating patients but can lead to overuse of medical services, which is also patient abuse.

Further removed from public awareness is the current practice of hospitals buying physician practices. In 1988, a Hamilton/KSA survey of six hundred hospitals reported that 18 percent of hospitals were buying physician practices.[3] Because hospitals purchase physician practices to increase or assure continuation of patient admissions from these physicians, incentives exist for questionable and inappropriate admissions when other hospitals would more likely be a physician's choice.

Also obscured from public view is the competition between hospital groups and physician groups over use of jointly owned new technology. When two or three hospitals work out a joint venture for a mobile magnetic resonance unit or a lithotripsy unit, physicians may also establish their own joint venture to provide the same services. Since only physicians order such services, and because physicians are not required to obtain Certificates of Need, they can control utilization and price.

These new challenges to the traditional ethical standards of medical care have been a response to external forces affecting the financing of medical services, from Medicare's prospective payment system, contract bidding, and discounted rates for hospitals, to fee screens, utilization reviews, and discounted fees for physicians. During the 1980s, the culture of medical care changed at a fundamental level, as it adapted to a new environment. Previously shared medical care values and beliefs are no longer totally realistic and acceptable in today's environment.

New Ethical Concerns

From the conception of the Hippocratic Oath to the creation of the Patient's Bill of Rights, ethical codes have defined the responsibilities and obligations toward patients of medicine and health care organizations. Current ethical concerns in medical care are different, however, from previous ethical issues. For example, when physicians make an investment, whether in the stock market or a joint venture, they expect to earn a profit from their investment. If the investment is in a publicly traded stock, personal decisions of the physician-stockholder will have no effect on dividends. In a local medical joint venture, a physician-investor can substantially affect a return on investment by ordering unnecessary tests and procedures and by referring patients to a medical service in which he or she is a shareholder.

In the not too distant past, physicians worked together to largely eliminate the unethical practices of ghost surgery (in which a surgeon unknown to the patient performs the operation) and fee-splitting (in which the surgeon submits a bill and then gives a portion of the payment to the attending physician for referring the case). The Medicare program further protected patient interests by prohibiting various forms of kickbacks and by defining fraud and abuse practices. In addition, hospitals adopted conflict of interest policies to prevent trustee and employee abuse of their authority. Still, some unethical corporate practices have escaped accountability.

The public view now emerging is that the traditional service motives of hospitals and physicians are being replaced by financial motives that put a provider's economic concerns ahead of their concern for patients. In the past, the public viewed medical care as a service to society, which only secondarily provided an economic benefit to physicians and hospitals. Today, patients are concerned that physicians and hospitals have placed their economic welfare ahead of the well-being of patients. This new reality is often reported in newspaper articles and reports of congressional testimony that have highlighted examples of excessive testing, unnecessary medical procedures, higher prices, and excessive profits, which are affecting the public's trust in medical care. However, the extent to which new joint ventures in medical care have abused the public interest is unknown.

Rationalizing Ethical Issues

The reasons used to justify investment in joint ventures vary from one hospital to another, and from one physician to another. The usual reasons cited by hospitals are the need to develop new revenue sources to offset Medicare and Medicaid payment reductions, to protect existing market share, or to expand local market share. Physicians explain that they enter into joint venture investments in order to provide higher quality service than previously available, respond to dissatisfaction with a similar hospital service, add a new medical service to the community, or develop new income sources because the economic future of medical practice is increasingly uncertain. Both physicians and hospitals have justified their investments as making good business sense, as being legal, and as being the same as commercial firms' investments in new business ventures. Overlooked and unmentioned is the traditional medical ethic that a patient's interest is primary and ahead of any personal interest of a physician or corporate interest of a hospital.

The current hospital and physician enthusiasm for joint ventures ignores society's long held view that medical care is more than a business. Society rightly expects a higher standard of responsibility and accountability from providers of medical care than from other businesses. The opportunity for a business to take advantage of a customer is typically limited by competition, requirements for honesty in advertising, and the buyer's knowledge of the product or service. In contrast, a physician exercises discretionary medical judgment for treatments and procedures, and charges for these services without patients being able to judge either necessity or price.

Both physicians and hospitals have a higher calling than business firms. Ethical physicians have a concern for the health and well-being of patients that is responsive to patients' individual needs and more important to the physician than the physician's personal needs. Ethical hospitals have a primary concern for the health status and well-being of their communities and patients, and a desire to be responsive to physician directives. The rush into new medical ventures in order to obtain additional revenue sources or as a competitive market strategy has modified these previous ethical standards in health care. In 1919, the founders of the hospital accreditation program were sufficiently concerned about medical ethics that they established the physician's relationship with the hospital as distinct from other hospital employees by requiring an organized, separate medical staff not subject to the control of the CEO, thus freeing doctors to exercise clinical judgment. The intention was to prevent patient care from being compromised by hospitals.

Often unrecognized are the differences in ethical standards for hospitals and physicians. Ethical conduct for a physician is defined as protecting and promoting the well-being of patients; they are not responsible for the financial success of hospitals, insurance carriers, or government medical programs. Hospitals have tougher ethical standards to meet, including fostering the well-being of both patients and the community, and survival of the corporation. The hospital cannot allow physicians to bankrupt the hospital while diagnosing and treating patients; therefore, as financial resources become more restricted and corporate survival is at stake, ethical conflicts between hospitals and physicians will arise.

Whether business relationships between hospitals and physicians are viewed as ethical or unethical depends on the ethical values of the individuals involved. For example, some hospital executives and physicians have justified investment in a variety of joint ventures by claiming that fee limitations for physicians and price caps for hospitals by Medicare, with utilization controls on both, have led to reduced incomes. Other observations have been one-sided: for instance, hospital executives have expressed the opinion that freestanding imaging centers are unethical because they are sponsored by physicians who are also members of the hospital's medical staff, and physicians have expressed the opinion that a hospital's efforts to stop the development of physician-sponsored imaging centers are unethical. Both views are smoke screens for justifying personal opinion.

Managed care programs sponsored by hospitals and physicians have been criticized by other physicians and hospital CEOs as unethical, based on the suspicion that in order to reduce expenses and increase profits hospitalized patients are discharged early or needed tests and medical procedures are not ordered. Allegations of unethical practices by joint ventures have been made to justify opposition to them, whether or not there is in fact any abuse of ethical standards. Many joint ventures may be completely ethical in the conduct of their affairs; nevertheless, they may be viewed as unethical by other hospital executives and physicians. Most hospitals and physicians are aware that ethical behavior is the bedrock of patient trust and essential to the public's belief that a patient's health and pocketbook will be protected. For joint ventures to avoid criticism, they must avoid even the appearance of unethical conduct.

The Impact of Revenue Restrictions

In the mid 1980s, a spurt of interest in finding new sources of revenue gave birth to Medicare's adoption of a prospective payment system based on diagnostic related groups, or DRGs, for reimbursing hospitals; a mandatory assignment program for physicians; and the use of maximum allowable actual cost methodology for nonparticipating physicians in the Part B fund of Medicare (which pays physicians). At about the same time, health insurance carriers began a significant effort to sponsor managed care programs, particularly HMOs and PPOs, using discounted hospital charges and physician fees.

Prior to the creation of these new programs, during the 1970s, only a few hospitals and physicians entered into a business relationship beyond a medical staff appointment. Today, there is widespread concern that financial limitations will continue to be tightened in the future, which will stimulate additional joint ventures. In the past, hospitals and physicians grudgingly accepted restrictive changes in payment systems and responded in a variety of ways to maintain existing income levels. As additional revenue restrictions are adopted in the future, pressure to deviate from ethical standards will increase.

With the upward spiral of medical care costs continuing, the stage is being set for drastic revenue limitations to bring costs under control. For hospitals and physicians to remain totally ethical in the future will require deep pockets. When politicians, bureaucrats, industry and business leaders, and insurance executives adopt new revenue and income restrictions, they will assume that hospitals and physicians will continue to place their economic and practice freedoms secondary to patient care responsibilities. However, as restrictions increase, more and more hospitals and physicians will question the price of being medically ethical.

In the current environment, hospitals and physicians are in a quandary about balancing patient interests with their tightening finances. When hospital revenue and physician income are significantly impacted, it is reasonable to expect corporate and personal interests to modify professional ethics. Ethical behavior is a two-way street and does not occur in a vacuum. For example, Medicare is again considering combining hospital and physician payments as a way to improve control of physician fees. Many health care professionals predict an enraged response if this plan is adopted.

The actions of the federal government, insurance carriers, and business have created an ethical dilemma for medical care. Each has defined and limited their responsibilities to the operational imperatives of their environment: the Medicare program sees its responsibility as paying the direct costs of care for the elderly and for its effect on the federal deficit; insurance carriers limit their responsibility to being competitive with other carriers; and business limits itself to being competitive in world markets. None of these viewpoints has been seriously concerned with the ultimate impact of policy decisions on the financial stability of hospitals and on physician incomes.

The gradual erosion of funding for medical indigence and the lack of availability of broad health insurance coverage should be of equal ethical concern to government, insurance carriers, and business. Instead, substantial portions of these responsibilities have been transferred by default to hospitals and physicians. Yet society still expects to receive needed medical care, even when payments to hospitals and physicians are inadequate, denied, or not available.

There is no demonstrable concern on the part of government and business for the financial well-being of medical care providers. This lack of fairness in their approaches to health care providers and in their attitudes toward the public's expectations for medical care creates an environment that encourages hospitals and physicians to offset revenue reductions through new business relationships. In a nutshell, utilitarianism has been the guiding principle, and equity for hospitals and physicians has been ignored. Increasingly coercive medical practice and a corporate environment have encouraged new business ventures and a commercial approach to medical care.

The Impact of Legislation

Unresponsive or irresponsible government and business policies do not justify either the appearance of unethical practice or its actual occurrence in medical care. At the very least, a joint venture may now create a public suspicion and raise questions about the extent to which patients can trust that medical services will be appropriate, necessary, and competitively priced. When medical relationships are established, a basic issue should be to assure an ethical operation that protects patient interests.

Quality medical care is premised on patients' trust of physicians, and on their belief that hospitals are trustworthy. Whenever unethical or questionable joint venture practices become public, all joint ventures become suspect—and public officials propose legislation to eliminate questionable practices. Such proposals are often poorly defined and may create unnecessary difficulties for medically ethical business relationships.

As hospital revenues shrink and physician fees are restricted, the incentive to consider joint ventures increases. Recent experience has shown that while a limited number of ventures have been profitable, many have not been a financial success. It is hoped that as operating experience increases, more ventures may become profitable. If new business partnerships between hospitals and physicians are necessary, then a way must be found to assure the public that these operations are ethical and will not compromise patient care and pocketbooks.

In 1985, Congress enacted Medicare fraud and abuse legislation to ensure a higher standard of ethical practice in medical care. In the 1989 session of Congress, an amended ethics bill for Medicare sponsored by Representative Stark was passed, with an effective date in 1992. The thrust of this legislation was to prohibit referrals to medical services in which a physician has an ownership interest, a move in the right direction, but the bill covered only Medicare patients, who do not account for the majority of referrals.

Current critics of medical practice ethics do not acknowledge that most hospitals and physicians have been sensitive to even the appearance of unethical behavior and have avoided involvement in business relationships. Both value their integrity more than their financial well-being. As the result of both existing and future restrictions on payments for medical services, ethical physicians and hospitals will incur large losses in revenues by their refusal to compromise their ethical values.

The existing environment allows business-oriented corporations and practitioners to take advantage of an unregulated medical marketplace for personal benefit, and abuses the ethically concerned who choose not to participate. The Medicare Fraud and

Abuse Act and the Stark ethics bill do not prohibit a range of potential ways in which creative medical entrepreneurs can exploit patients.

Current ethical precepts that guide medical care providers are in conflict with their income expectations as revenues for patient services are decreased. By far, hospitals and physicians strive to be ethical in their patient relationships and will struggle to continue to do so. However, adhering to ethical medical standards is not the totality of the ethics of physicians and hospitals. Providing medical care is only one dimension of an individual's ethical conduct: physicians are also parents, citizens, community-participants, and a host of other roles. Hospitals as corporations have a multiplicity of obligations: at all levels of government, to the judicial system, to commercial involvements, and as models of the corporate community in a city.

The intersection of multiple ethical expectations and the effort to find ways to accommodate conflicting ethical behavior may require a shift in ethical standards. As limited payments for medical care services continue to spread, modifications of traditional medical ethics can be expected to occur. Traditional medical ethical standards will be sidestepped or gradually be modified to accommodate new realities.

The basic issue is whether change in ethical standards will occur by external forces or be driven internally by medical practitioners. In the present medical care environment, further revenue and income limitations will create new incentives to modify ethical standards. Changes in standards will be limited by the principle that only when physicians' discretionary judgments about medical care remain the physicians' decisions can adequate medical care for patients be provided.

The difficulty of protecting a physician's discretionary decision making is that such discretion provides an opportunity to exploit the economic freedom enjoyed by physicians. Joint ventures, Medicare, and managed care provide financial vehicles for profit at the expense of medical ethics. If traditional ethical standards of medical care are important to society, these standards must be protected from all forms of abuse. Current competitive, financial, and regulatory practices create ethical dilemmas in protecting patient interests. Government, insurance carriers, physicians, and hospitals separately and collectively compromise patient care, both indirectly and overtly, by their existing policies. To continue to maintain traditional medical ethics requires the establishment of severe restraints on existing corporate and regulatory practices. The kinds of restraints needed to eliminate compromise of patient care would reduce medical practice incomes and would likely encourage more overt price increases where loopholes exist in the regulatory and insurance company pricing mechanisms. The restraints needed would be a total ban on interlocking corporate physician relationships and on physician-group-to-physician-group investment arrangements.

Enactment of legislation to prevent joint arrangements at a time when federal policy is further restricting medical care revenues would further exacerbate existing revenue limitations on hospitals and physicians. If an accreditation program were chosen as the control mechanism, other difficulties would occur. For an accreditation process to be meaningful, an accreditation organization would need the public's confidence that its programs were objective and meaningful, and that certification would assure ethical standards of operation. However, standards for making these judgments are equivocal. Clinical standards of appropriate use are affected by a patient's condition, by the preliminary diagnosis, and by the medical knowledge of the referring physician.

Excessive profits are also elusive to define and are affected by fluctuating volumes, markups of tests and procedures, and marketing variables. At best, expert judgment would only identify gross abuses. If arbitrary guides were used, they would most likely be either too strict or too loose. An annual medical and financial audit by a respected independent organization could be a useful solution, but no organization that is capable of providing such services has public acceptance.

Conclusions

The widespread development of joint ventures is a serious indication that the medical culture is in a process of change. Previously held ethical values and beliefs are being attenuated by internal and external forces as the medical enterprise seeks to adapt to income limitations. Medical ideals worth striving for are being modified by personal and corporate concerns.

The reality of rapidly increasing medical care costs will sooner or later force the adoption of a new approach to providing medical care. The most likely development will be either a fixed fee system of paying physicians or the total elimination of fee-for-service medical practice. Along with these changes, hospitals will be targets for major policy decisions that will institute either reduced DRG payments or the adoption of a per-patient-day fixed payment system.

It is therefore probable that previously held ethical values and beliefs will continue to be attenuated. The traditional ethical primacy of patient interests will gradually be replaced by a value system that expands the welfare of society at the expense of the individual. The traditional ethical medical point of view will slowly disappear as medicine and institutional programs of care are changed by competitive marketplace economics that are progressively financially untenable.

Notes
1. "$70 Consulting Fee Paid by a Texas Hospital to Physician for Each Patient Admitted." *The Wall Street Journal,* February 28, 1989.
2. "Average Number of Tests Ordered by Physician Investor Was 6.23 Tests per Patient and 3.76 for Non-physician Investors." *The Wall Street Journal,* March 1, 1989.
3. *The Wall Street Journal,* March 1, 1989.

Part Two

Managed Care

Chapter Six

Capitation

The Wave of the Future?

Richard L. Johnson

Hospitals and physicians are rushing headlong into forming larger and larger provider units in the belief that increasing size and numbers in economic units or affiliated organizations is the only route to survival under capitation. The driving force is the belief that if a local health care provider controls enough units of service, the managed care plan will be forced to offer the integrated provider a reasonable contract. If the hospital and the associated physicians are well-regarded in public opinion, the plan may feel compelled to contract with the strong, large, well-established provider if it is to be successful in marketing its products in that community.

The basic assumption being made by health care providers is that capitation will be the dominant form of prepaying for health care coverage and, like it or not, providers must be prepared to compete to provide services in this environment. Fee-for-service payments to physicians, per diem rates, or discounted charges to hospitals are seen as rapidly dying ways of paying providers. Climbing onto the new bandwagon is seen as the path to survival in the new economic era. Capitation is attractive to the federal government, which pays for Medicare; to state governments, which pay a large share of the Medicaid program; and to employers, who pay health premiums on behalf of their employees.

Perspectively, the federal government is eyeing capitation as the way of clamping the lid on the steady escalation of Medicare payments to health care providers. To limit future occurrences of the unanticipated rises that have occurred over the years, federal legislators have initiated a number of activities, starting with the cost freeze in the Nixon administration, followed by the voluntary cost containment program of the Carter years, the adoption of DRGs in the 1980s, and finally, the capitation bill under the Clinton administration. Up to this point, federal legislators have concluded that providers have failed to contain health care costs, and they believe that what is needed is a federal program that caps Medicare expenditures through federally determined capitation rates and, at the same time, shifts the financial risks to the providers.

State governments have been equally concerned about the Medicaid program, which has chewed up an ever-increasing percentage of state government revenues. Governors in a number of states have initiated legislation and implemented programs with the same objectives as those of the federal government, shifting the financial risk to the providers and away from the government. As a result of financial distress, both federal and state governments are turning to capitation as the way of alleviating their health care dilemmas.

Employers also have had concerns about the annual escalation they have experienced in employee health care premiums. This acceleration has led employers to seriously consider switching their coverage to managed care plans that offer capitation. One of the major problems employers experience is that in making a decision in favor of capitation they limit their employees' and their families' selection of physicians and hospitals. This is troublesome to many employers because they believe that employees should not be so restricted and would thus prefer to avoid such constraints. Given the option of free choice versus limited choice, most employers would prefer free choice for their employees, if annual premium increases would rise no faster than the consumer price index.

The Gatekeeper System

For a number of years there has been criticism of the traditional method of payments to both hospitals and physicians in which the episode of illness is unhooked from any economic consequence to the patient. The argument has been made that this gives the patient a blank check from the medical care system and therefore leads to abuse. To create controls on the use of health care resources, prepayment carriers introduced the concepts of deductibles and coinsurance. The thought behind the creation of these methods was that if patients have to pay for initial visits to physicians (the gatekeepers), they will be judicious in deciding when to make an appointment. In the same view, coinsurance was seen as a brake on overutilization of health care resources, particularly for hospitalizations.

Eventually, deductibles and coinsurance became standard provisions in many prepayment contracts. What had started out as a way to control excessive use of the health care system turned out to have an additional value to prepayment organizations. By increasing deductibles and coinsurance payments, carriers were able to protect their profit margins. Even when the services of health care providers rose at a faster rate than the consumer price index, the prepayment organizations found they could juggle premium increases, deductibles, and coinsurance so as to cushion the impact on employers of annual rate adjustments.

Eventually, this system ran into competitive problems and began to lose subscribers to managed care plans that contracted with health care providers for services on a discounted fee basis or that offered capitated payment plans. By relying on gatekeepers, capitated plans were able to achieve significant reductions in the utilization of hospitals and specialists, which turned out to be economically important. Hospital care represents 40 percent of all of the costs of the health care system and is by far the most expensive aspect of health care. As a result of its early successes, capitation became the darling of those who pay for care on a group basis.

Capitation is attractive because its cornerstone is the use of primary care physicians as gatekeepers of entry into the medical care system. The capitation system is designed and operated to prevent the patient from making a decision to see a specialist as a self-referral, even though it may be evident to a reasonable person which type of specialist should be seen. The cost to the patient for going outside of the system is having to pay the full or a partial amount of the charges rendered—an economic penalty. Usually unknown to the patient is that gatekeepers may be rewarded with bonuses at the end of the year for keeping patients away from specialists by providing as much of the care as possible themselves. Such a system is open to manipulation by the managed care plan and primary care physicians. For example, by decreasing the monthly capitated rate paid to the gatekeeper and increasing the amount available for year-end bonuses, the gatekeeper physician may be influenced to reduce specialist referrals.

Shifting the Risk

Overlooked in capitation is that the episode of illness still remains unhooked from any economic consequence to patients. Capitation substitutes the gatekeeper physician as the surrogate for the patient as decision maker. In doing so, the managed care plan obtains a benefit in addition to the one of reduced utilization. By contracting with primary care physicians, most of the financial risk is shifted to the physicians. In return for a fixed monthly payment, the primary care physician is obligated to provide medical care to whatever extent it is either desired or needed by the patients covered by the plan.

The managed care plan has the same desire to shift financial risk from the managed care plan to the hospital. The hospital may be offered one capitated rate per month for all of its services. This is a desirable method of payment for the carrier since it shifts nearly all of the financial risk to the providers, hospitals, and primary care physicians, with specialist usage controlled by the gatekeepers. If hospital fees are not capitated, the fallback position of the plan is to pay a fixed amount per case based on diagnosis, or to pay a fixed amount per day of hospital care. The least desirable method of payment for the plan is to pay a discounted percentage of the charges billed to a patient.

By capitating fees for all of the providers of health care services on a contractual basis, the managed care plan receives many advantages. By shifting the risks for services to the providers, the managed care plan becomes a conduit for funds, taking off up front all of the monies not obligated to providers. By shifting the risk to providers, the managed care plan has far more control over its own expenses. It can devote its major efforts to marketing, paying claims, and monitoring physician performance. In the event that gatekeeper physicians refer too few patients to specialists and therefore have poor patient outcomes, or if, conversely, too many patients are referred to specialists, the managed care plan may replace physicians. The control of the economics lies in either changing providers or securing performance adherence to the carrier's norms.

Selecting Partners

The economics of health care now dominate the thinking of both the providers of services and those who pay for the care. This has led physicians and hospitals to scramble to find partners with which to merge, consolidate, or affiliate. The loose informality that has long characterized health care provider relationships is quickly ending. The external threat from managed care is driving physicians and hospitals into common organizational structures.

Coming to terms with the need to become ever larger economic entities is difficult for both physicians and hospitals. Neither group really wants to do so, but they see no alternative because they are fearful of the consequences of remaining freestanding. Accommodation to this change is difficult and fraught with emotion, untried relationships, and concern about making mistakes in the choice of partners. There is a fear that longstanding "truths" will turn out to be nothing more than working assumptions that have to be laid aside and replaced with new ideas that must be embraced before being fully understood. The future lacks clarity and is only dimly recognized, yet managed care pressures seem to require adopting partners without fully understanding the trends of the future.

These hospital/physician partnerships are being formed out of economic necessity brought about by the threat of massive capitation. Since capitation goes hand in hand with growth in competition, the higher the percentage of the population covered by capitation, the more intense will be the competition among health care providers. Capitation pits hospitals against hospitals, primary care physicians against specialists, and specialists against specialists. Carried to an extreme degree, capitation can become a destructive force in a community. Surviving in an intensely competitive environment requires abandoning the traditional values of giving back to the community the benefits resulting from a profitable operation. Of necessity, the focus is on outdoing the competitor institutions and on aligning physicians with health care organizations. Leveraging managed care contracts becomes the "only game in town." Social values take a back seat to competition. In the emerging economic era, those who cling to traditions that are no longer viable will find failure rather than success. Important as they were, the cultural values associated with being nonprofit will be replaced as capitation forces hospitals to reexamine their value systems.

As capitation increases, the competitive forces become stronger and stronger. Hospitals believe that to offset this pressure they must become larger and larger economic entities encompassing both hospital and physician services. The alternative is to be taken over by a larger, more dominant health care provider. The hospital must assess what it needs to do. The competition is not just other hospitals but, more importantly, the managed care plans operating in the area. Managed care is likely to play a decisive role in shaping the health care delivery system of the future.

Advantages and Disadvantages of Capitation

The rationale behind putting together all the elements needed for a delivery system into a regional presence is to force managed care plans to contract for services because of the importance of the delivery system in the area. The purpose of a delivery system is to capture as much of the prepayment (capitated) revenues as possible. In the rush to respond to the imperatives of capitation, the public may fail to appreciate the limitations of this method, which include the following:

- Capitation substitutes a limited list of contracted primary care physicians from which the subscriber must choose.
- Capitation prevents self-referral to a specialist.
- Capitation puts no economic risk on patients as long as they stay within the system.
- Capitation substitutes a primary care physician's economic decisions for those of the patient.
- Capitation shifts the economic risk from the managed care plan to the provider.

- Capitation typically obtains most of its information on the way the system is working "after the fact"—that is, after the service has been rendered, when the managed care plan is paying claims.
- Capitation primarily provides a conduit for managed care plans to receive and distribute funds, and to serve as a repository for data.
- Capitation does not rehook the episode of illness to economic consequences for the patient.
- Capitation leads to an increase in the use of physician extenders—individuals with less training than physicians, such as physician assistants, nurses, and so on.
- Capitation leads to a statistical mind-set of managing populations, not of providing care to individuals.

The literature of the health care field tends to highlight the average number of inpatient days per one thousand people. The impression is created that the lower the number, the more appropriate the care is, because less money is being spent on the most expensive component of health care. Does this really mean, for example, that a managed care plan that provides two hundred inpatient days of care per one thousand people is providing more appropriate care than one that provides three hundred inpatient days of care?

The use of restricted lists of primary care physicians, specialists, and hospitals for capitation not only leads to patients being concerned about not having freedom of choice from among the providers, but physicians have become fearful of being left out. This has resulted in the development in some states of legislation known as *willing provider laws*. These laws mandate that each managed care company open its provider panels to any licensed physician willing to comply with the practice guidelines adopted by the managed care company. The purpose of this law is to ensure competition in the marketplace for physician services. Faced with this legislation, managed care plans are concerned that such competition will happen and their ability to successfully negotiate low professional fees will be destroyed because they will not be able to control the flow of patients. Managed care plans are concerned that without an ability to control the number of contract physicians, they will not be able to generate sufficient patient volume to be financially attractive to individual participating physicians.

Because of the inherent shortcomings of capitation, there is a need to develop a system that rehooks the episode of illness with economic consequences to the patient. If this can be accomplished, it may be possible to achieve lower utilizations and lower expenditures and thereby enable lower premium costs to the employees.

Capitation does offer some advantages. These include the following:

- Capitation integrates physicians and hospitals into a common delivery system.
- Capitation offers one price for both hospital and physician services.
- Capitation reduces excess usage of the health care system.
- Capitation establishes clinical pathways and outcome measures of performance.
- Capitation encourages development of wellness programs.

In communities in which capitation is in competition with traditional methods of prepayment, the providers find themselves with mixed incentives. Both hospitals and physicians tend to give preference to those patients covered by fee-for-service prepayment plans, because each unit of service rendered leads to additional revenue. Under capitation, the amount of money received remains constant, even if the units of service increase.

Capitation is a competitive model only insofar as providers of service are concerned. It is not a competitive model for users because the users do not make economic choices; the options are left to the primary care physician serving as the gatekeeper. A true marketplace competitive model would put the users of the health care system in the position of making economic choices. Yet, it is unrealistic to expect patients to make these economic choices without having full knowledge of their medical consequences.

Conclusions

It can be predicted that ultimately the limitations of capitation will be publicly recognized. When disillusionment sets in, the public will commence searching for a new strategy that is more responsive to their needs, which they will define as freedom to select their own physicians and hospital, as well as greater convenience. They will desire a plan with fewer rules and a system for assisting them in making economic/medical decisions. As the discontent grows among participants in capitation plans, employers will be open to alternatives that permit employees and dependents to select their own physicians, as long as premium increases do not exceed the rate of inflation. It is to be expected that employers will turn away from capitation to a true competitive model in which the resulting savings will directly benefit those who buy the coverage and not accrue to the benefit of the managed care plan.

When the public recognizes that the artificial barriers of capitation plans are not in their best interests, they will turn to a system that puts patients' interests first. The lesson yet to be learned is that a truly competitive marketplace model can work in health care by providing a system that assists patients in making decisions. The system does not have to rely on a gatekeeper whose decisions are measured by how little patients use the health care system. Experience has shown that the public can be trusted to make the appropriate decisions when given support in understanding the economic and medical factors that come into play, and when empowered with the responsibility for their own well-being.

Chapter Seven

Power and New Economic Relationships

Montague Brown

Power over and control of America's vast medical care infrastructure are being shifted away from traditional providers, especially hospitals and physicians.[1] They are going to business firms whose guiding principles are ill-understood by America's health policy elite, hospital boards, and physicians. The benefits (profits, growth, power) are being captured not by patients and buyers but by managed care firms and insurers, who seek control over patients and use that control to pressure providers to decrease their use of resources in treating patients and to do what they do for lower prices.

Real and Profound Change

Has there really been a shift in the balance of power? To see where power is shifting to, follow the money trail. A lead story by George Anders in *The Wall Street Journal* chronicled this shift.[2] Anders chronicled an earnings surge among health maintenance organizations (HMOs) seeking to grow, cash reserves in the millions, and an industry segment that has pushed down its costs by getting

Note: A version of this chapter was published under the title "Managed Care: Power and New Economic Relationships," in *Physician Executive,* December 1995. Used here with permission of American College of Physician Executives.

provider discounts and by closely managing care given to consumers while at the same time keeping prices to buyers as high as possible.

The story of managed care today is about power, about ownership of the infrastructure, and about the soul of health care; it is not yet about consumer benefits. Those who see ultimate consumer benefits from this slippery slope we are on today must be assuming that once the new regime is in power and has monopoly control (market share in the range of 50 to 100 percent) it will operate as a benevolent dictator and not as a normal profit-oriented business. Too many of these seers probably still believe in the tooth fairy. The first priority of a business is to serve its shareholders' interest in growing wealth. To do this, it must master market demand; it may only incidentally lower cost or confer major new benefits on consumers. If consumer benefit is to be derived from business ownership and control of medicine it will be necessary to understand how business operates so that effective strategies can be developed to ensure patient safety and sophistication and clout for buyers.

The transformation of health into a business-run operation is rapid, accelerating, and powerful. "While Congress remains silent, health care transforms itself," said Erik Eckholm in *The New York Times*.[3] Eckholm chronicled the transformation going on in managed care, the merging of insurers, and the expansion of market share by nontraditional organizations. According to Arnold S. Relman, editor emeritus of the *New England Journal of Medicine,* "There never has been a time in the history of American medicine when the independence and autonomy of medical practitioners was as uncertain as it is now."[4] The transformation is about power and control, which translate into money. Money has always been the game of Wall Street, entrepreneurs, and business, but now, perhaps, it is foremost the game of health care. The role of money in health care is little understood and often blindly maligned, and its force in the field is therefore grossly underestimated.

Tom Weil[5] made a strong case that capitation, managed care, and regionalization are simply new names for old concepts put forward, at times successfully, by medical and social reformers over the past fifty years. Mergers, managed care, regional systems and the like are based on models that were developed by social engineers (medical care organization practitioners and teachers, royal commissions, and others). The same concepts of organization are now found appealing by capitalist conservatives. The behavior of managed care firms, including not-for-profit firms, fits the profit-seeking business model much more than the earlier social models that prompted reform efforts to develop regional systems and pre-paid group practices.

Organizational concepts conceived by socialists and run along the lines of a modern state enterprise have little or nothing in common with the modern, capitalist business enterprise. Conversely, as in the modern state, control in capitalist businesses is often in the hands of a few people (with management usually part of that group) who use the power of the corporation to further their own goals. For the private enterprise, the goal is generally wealth, and for the state enterprise executive and power groups, it is lifelong control.

Capitation: A Quantum Leap away from Tradition

Traditional health insurance was grafted onto a World War II wartime wage and price control policy that banned wage increases. Employers bought Blue Cross and Blue Shield coverage for their employees, which paid providers their charges or cost plus, and when costs rose Blue Cross and Blue Shield passed along the increases to an undemanding customer. Private insurers followed in the 1960s with similar packages, but also with a marketing strategy of cherry picking low-risk customers while paying providers the same rates, which resulted in higher profits. This form of insurance guaranteed price escalation, so by the 1970s, inflation of health care costs was twice as high as the consumer price index, a condition that is currently moderating only mildly.

Indemnity coverage (paying dollar amounts rather than per unit of service) basically encourages resource use, multiple referrals, and higher cost. Providers are paid only after encounters and the performance of services. Managed care and capitation are designed to correct this fundamental flaw that drives up cost. Managed care seeks to limit the use of resources by consumers by prohibiting and controlling the circumstances in which patients make use of physicians. Capitation, and various other forms of paying fixed prices to providers, is used to give a financial incentive to providers to lower resource use—or lose money. Providers are paid fixed amounts in advance of service or fixed amounts for given conditions, without respect to whether more or less is done.

Many providers still wonder just what capitation is and how far it can be extended. Simply put, a capitation is an amount of money offered to a vendor for a particular type of service or good that may be needed for a defined population. The amount of money *likely* to be needed by any provider, specialist, or vendor (say, a staple manufacturer) can be calculated from existing massive insurance files on millions of cases. Information on likely use is first determined according to such variables as age, sex, preexisting conditions, medical practice styles in the region, and other known determinants of need, and the results are then projected forward for a given population. If the databases are large enough, all medical specialists can be included among those paid capitated fees. Even vendors are being asked to accept capitated payments. (In fact, many specialists have not yet been asked to accept capitation, and some who have accepted it say it does not work—that is, it does not reduce waste. There is some doubt in my own mind that even HMOs or employers feel they have sufficiently benefited from the gross waste in the system to make it necessary to capitate. That, of course, is another story outside the scope of this chapter.)

In one respect, insurance payments have always been capitated. When a carrier quotes a yearly rate, it must operate within that rate for the year. In the past, raising prices to consumers merely meant that when costs exceeded premiums, the premium was raised at year-end to recoup the loss and get ahead of the usual increases of the next year. Anyone who watches such increases will remember business complaints about 30 to 40 percent increases in one year; that was catch-up pricing.

The United States is now in a fixed-price, capitation market for health care. This is not the future. It is the present, and the situation has many implications for who will dominate, control, and ultimately dictate the values of health care providers and institutions.

Public Policy Endorses Managed Care

Although many of the ideas discussed here were put forth by both Clinton and the Republicans, these ideas were truly idolized by conservatives. While prepaid group practice might have originated as a socialist idea, it is not seen by conservatives as a socialist reform. The economic system in the United States is market capitalism, and it rewards businesses based on who can offer the best price. "Socialist-type reform is dead, but capitalism is harder to fight," says Bob Burnett, a doctor from California.[6] If by fighting managed care American medicine seeks to roll back the clock, the battle will indeed be difficult, perhaps impossible, before the structural revolution is beyond reversal.

In America, policy shifts in disjointed, incremental ways—a lesson learned again in the Clinton health care debate. It is thus unlikely that any significant policy shifts will occur before predictions on likely shifts in ownership, power, and control take hold.

Those who fear that the business ethic and profit motive might—indeed, are likely to—destroy the social mission of the hospital and undermine the tradition of medicine will want to try and stop this trend. Those who are leading the change are equally convinced that there is much more fat in the system and profits to be made before any ill overtakes their efforts. Those in search of profits can also use this pitch to justify why they can no longer lower prices to consumers without jeopardizing patient care.

The forces undergirding the change are too embedded in the social and health care fabric to be altered before a major transformation of the system occurs. Since Medicare and Medicaid were enacted, with the promise that health care was or would soon become a right, Wall Street dollars have fueled a revolution in financing not-for-profit, public, and investor-owned hospitals and, in more recent years, major HMOs. The discipline of watching the hospital balance sheet through the eyes of philanthropy and community giving has now been completely replaced with a green-eyeshade approach that looks first and foremost at the financial indicators used by financial rating agencies. Decisions about pricing and programs are screened carefully for their impact on financial ratios. This is justified by even the most conservative socially oriented institutions. The slogan used is, "We must do well to do good." Financially weak institutions simply do not survive.

It might be reasonable to ask whether or not the revolution in ownership and control of hospitals that has emerged during the past twenty years is a result of traditional thinking or new, market-oriented forces.[7] As Weil argued, regionalization, health systems, and alliances are the end results of effective organization and rationalization of health care service delivery. Although it is easy to agree—to say yes, that is true—it is profoundly incorrect to then assume that these terms mean the same to profit-oriented equity- and debt-market financiers that they meant to generations of medical care organizations, governmental commissions, and bureaucrats.

Lowering Costs

When entrepreneurial capitalists look at the Kaiser Foundation Plan and similar prepaid group practices, they see opportunities to produce medical services at lower cost, but they do not think first of turning these lower costs into refunds or lower prices for the community. They see the difference between their lower costs and the costs and prices of competitors, and based on this difference they arrive at a price to the consumer that maximizes profits to the firm. When researchers look at profit-seeking organizations and find that these institutions can thrive merely by raising their prices, not by becoming more efficient, the researchers are aghast and think that profit seeking cannot lower cost. The world I see is not so simple. The following example of how things might actually work is instructive.

A government-owned provider that actually lowers cost would also need to lower taxes or find new ways to spend the "dividend" arising from the difference between cost and prices. My own experience with governments is that they spend surpluses and rarely, if ever, return unused funds or call for lower taxes. A for-profit firm has no such problem with returning surplus in the form of dividends. The for-profit firm will price a service to beat the competition, but it will never merely lower prices to where they will just cover costs. One only has to watch drug pricing to see how this works. New drugs are priced on the basis of the value they deliver to customers, not on what it costs to produce them. Governments tend to price based on cost, while businesses price based on what the market will pay for acceptable substitutes for the product or service. This difference between public agencies and those organized to produce private profits is profound. Many public-health and social-policy scholars tend to evaluate health care on the basis of whether access is extended, costs are limited, or quality is greatly enhanced. While large drops in cost may be technically feasible, neither not-for-profit organizations nor governmental units nor for-profit concerns are likely to declare a public benefit dividend. All have their reasons, and to some extent they are the same. Those who are successful at what they do generally want to keep the reward.

Many of the regionalization concepts were developed for public policies that assumed a public benefit would accrue from lowered cost, improved access, and/or higher quality. When such models are used by profit-seeking institutions, they generally produce lower cost, improved access, and higher quality for consumers *if and only if there is greater profit to the producer for the effort, and the profit precedes any benefits to consumers.* What is worse is that it is not clear that any benefit will be passed on to consumers without a greatly empowered consumer or buyer federation, or without a greatly expanded and empowered government watchdog, even stronger than the watchdog considered by the Clinton administration in 1993 and 1994.

How do such bald assertions about profit-seeking behavior fit with the data? Some data suggest that managed care plans produce a very small cost advantage.[8] An article in *The Wall Street Journal* notes the large cash reserves and growth of HMOs.[9] Profit-making firms will price their products at levels carefully designed to be sufficiently attractive to consumers; that is, they will price lower than indemnity coverage, but they will only need to go low enough to get buyers to switch to their products. If competitors' prices remain higher, firms never need to go much lower to get or keep business. This type of behavior leads to only modest lowering of prices, and to the big cash buildups, mergers, and acquisitions that characterize the health care industry today.

There is a public benefit to be derived from low-cost delivery models, but how fast and how far prices to consumers will actually be reduced depends very much on how fast competitors adapt to lower-cost methods of doing business. Only when competitive choices are available at even lower cost will innovators go back to the well for cost savings to the consumer. The thesis presented here argues that those who can produce at lower cost can gain market share and increased profits with only nominal cuts in pricing, and that, barring increased competition, they have very little incentive to push prices down further. The kinds of cash positions reported in *The Wall Street Journal* are consistent with this concept.

The Role of HMOs

It is widely known that most of the new HMOs seek price discounts from providers in return for favorable referral policies. As long as they can get such discounts, they have little reason to push hard for more efficiency from providers. When the discounts no longer give the HMO a competitive price edge, they seek further concessions on utilization and other cost features. In markets where traditional providers resist managed care, it is possible to see years of no change, with managed care options growing slowly and showing only modest price leadership.

In fact, HMOs do not even need to push themselves to become substantially more cost-efficient when the market offers little competition for even the most modest reforms. This lack of competition could easily account for the fact that HMOs never seem to get around to price cutting below the entry-level fees that differentiate them from indemnity and PPO products.

It is not inconsistent for political conservatives or Wall Street investors to argue that prepaid group practices and all the modern forms of managed care can bring costs down. What they fail to add is the parallel fact that this promise will only result in lower cost to consumers if and when providers are forced to actually cut costs (by using least-cost methods) in order to meet competitive prices in the marketplace. Some variation on this behavior occurs in not-for-profit and government agencies, so it is not unique for investor-owned institutions to do this. Managed care exhibits the same type of behavior.

Will business and government buyers continue to buy at prices that could be brought down if more pressure were put on HMOs to bring them down? Given the knowledge that businesses have about how profit maximization behavior occurs, and given the major news reports on profitability and cash reserves, it seems likely that business will seek better deals. HMOs will provide such deals only *if and when* buyers can find lower-cost alternatives to what HMOs offer. For some businesses this will mean renting networks, building their own managed care products, or finding ways to contract around the HMOs. However, as the networks vertically integrate with providers and settle into market shares that limit competition, the ability of buyers to find such options will decline.

Insurers can no longer count on buyers to increase payments to account for increases in expenses. Buyers are seeking relief from annual premium increases they have been experiencing over the last few years. It is no secret that insurers, including the Blue Cross plans, are trying to shift all of their business into managed care. All managed care plans start out with minimal change in the status quo of medical practice. Price discounts are given while providers raise overall prices to other consumers, thus adding to the burdens of cost shifting. Some truly weird things have happened as a result of such practices. In Virginia, Blue Cross was charged with getting kickbacks when its negotiated price was less than the deductible paid by the patient, thus creating a windfall for the hospital which was then rebated to Blue Cross. In New York, a Blue Cross plan was charged with having individual contract holders subsidize large employers who got discounts. All of this activity has come under the rubric of managed care, some of it in HMOs. All of it (in both for-profit and not-for-profit firms) is consistent with profit maximizing behavior, and none of it matches the dreams and aspirations of any expert on medical care organization who for years might have advocated such organizational arrangements to improve access and lower cost for medical care.

The underlying paradigm in the managed care approach to health care is profit making, not community benefit maximizing. One can only wonder whether there ever has been any attempt by the industry to roll back prices and reduce costs to the community; the opposite seems to be the case. If there has been any discipline on cost to consumers it has been the rhetoric of "we can moderate cost escalation, but not cut cost." Only the boldest providers claim that the overall expenditures on medical care can actually be cut while broadening access to the uninsured.

Will modern HMOs ever pay off in lower costs? The answer must be that it depends on the competition. HMOs already beat traditional group and fee-for-service arrangements, and do very well against provider-dominated PPOs. The question itself might be better put by asking whether the status quo or some major regulatory scheme might be a better approach. Clearly, the HMOs, and modern managed care in general, do a bit better than the unfettered, noncompetitive indemnity approaches to cost containment. The nation benefits from vastly improved technology and world-class levels of specialized professional sophistication, which result in large part from the free-flowing cash coming from indemnity payments to ever-growing health insurance accounts.

Government tends to enrich the status quo when governmental controls are enhanced. Moderate growth in cost occurs, but never accompanied by any fundamental change. "Never" is not too strong a word for what happens. Medicare promised to never interfere with fee-for-service medical relations between patients and physicians, but that attitude changed so much in twenty-five years that it is hard to discern just when the promise fell and new forces took over. Conversely, while pricing certainly changed, there is still ample evidence of government reluctance to explicitly abandon this promise. Governments do not voluntarily lower taxes when costs are cut. Bureaucrats and vendors have a mutual interest in growing their share of the gross domestic product pie—unfortunately for both taxpayers and patients.

Do Options Exist?

If governments keep inflating taxes, rents, and health care costs, it might be reasonable to ask where in this gloom there might be some hope (for consumers, not HMOs or other providers). Investors price to the market and keep efficiency gains for profit. Hospitals and physicians clearly prefer to enjoy their current modes of doing business and will only yield to change under special circumstances.

Three approaches to getting solid community benefit and consumer cost savings are possible. The first approach is to get an enlightened governing body to insist on community benefit rather than institutional aggrandizement. Physicians and executives who get rewarded for growth will not easily yield to such ideas.

The second mode of change requires governmental "action with bite," which in this scenario would mean tough regulations, bureaucrats losing their jobs if costs do not come down, and politicians not getting elected if good things do not happen for the consumer. I am not optimistic that these things can be accomplished without major structural reforms in Congress, such as term limits, a balanced budget amendment, and the easing of civil service rules to make firing easier. The country is going in precisely the opposite direction today.

The third option is for buyers to keep pressing managed care companies for discounts and lower prices. This requires encouraging competition among modes of care, and it undoubtedly requires choices among providers and HMOs—something that will not exist if more markets are merged, effectively lessening the likelihood of competition.

Of all of the forces that might push down costs and prices to consumers, an informed buyer is most likely to make this happen. The informed buyer will have to push beyond price discounts that allow for cost shifting. He or she will push for business and government to embrace lower-cost methods of taking care of people and lower prices to reflect this lower cost. Business and government must seek better value, and use all their market power to achieve it.

At this point, the best method for lowering cost with some quality controls is prepaid group practice and similar HMOs. The best way to lower prices is to engage in more aggressive and informed buying. Buying right should reward high-quality low-cost producers with volume. Teachers would, I suspect, be aghast at the current market-oriented version of their concepts. Conversely, they would see that in many markets the promise of profit has achieved changes that previously were not readily available because of the traditional barriers to doing the right thing for the public good.

Pros and Cons of the Current Course

In a system that stresses cost, there is great risk that quality will eventually suffer—or as one orthopedist told me, he gets out the lower-quality "Medicare" prosthesis for those who cannot pay enough to cover the cost of the higher-quality device. This cost-driven behavior may not be in the patient's best interest. Of course, a case can be made for varying quality to allow patients to choose varying price levels for their care. Under a capitation plan, or any other tightly managed care system, quality and ultimate consumer benefit are at greater risk because financial incentives stress low cost and improved profits, not maximization of efforts on the consumer's behalf no matter what the level of cost-benefit expectation.

Weak providers will be pushed out of business. Perhaps worse, some of these providers will be those who provide most of their service to the poor. This is happening now, and the potential for it is being used by many interest groups, administrators, and boards throughout the nation to justify their business-like approach to pricing and profit making in their institutions.

Another casualty of today's managed care may be specialists. Not only will specialists be in less demand, but the specialists who opt early for managed care roles and their cost-consciousness may indeed not be the very best. We could also see the demise of subspecialty medicine. If my informants from England are correct, some specialties, like dermatology, have never thrived in an environment oriented to primary care. This loss of specialists might be one of the greatest costs of changing to a system that promotes profit and low cost over application of knowledge to patient needs.

Closely related to this loss of specialists is the still-small segment of the medical profession tied into the controlling and managing elements of the managed care movement. Many of the financially oriented managers and owners think that they can buy a bit of expertise from physicians, codify their methods, and turn the work over to nurses, clerks, and computers. We will never get fundamental and meaningful managed care without the unqualified support of, and without leadership from, the best professionals in every major discipline.[10]

Clearly, one change—a loss to some, a gain to others—is the shift during the past two decades of health care leadership from alignment with medicine's service orientation to alignment with business interests. An underlying principle that is inadequately stressed is the prime responsibility of health service governance and management to balance the health needs of the community with the economic realities of generating sufficient revenues to effectively and efficiently deliver the services required by the residents of the community. One of the major reasons that reform is needed is that providers have failed to move toward modes of care that recognize affordability as an important criterion for sustained support of any social service, including medicine. But this change in thinking about the field occurred before there was an affordability crisis.

After Medicare was passed, the need was truly great for capital to expand and modernize to meet the expected growth in demand for medical care. In order to modernize and expand, voluntary and public institutions began to rely on bond-market financing; even the most venerable institutions began to be managed with a sharp eye on financial performance. This reliance on public financing forever changed the industry. The requirement to manage by the numbers in order to get financing in the future brought more and more financially oriented administrators into the field and more businesspeople onto boards, and more and more boards judged performance with a sharp eye to meeting Wall Street ratios. No one should doubt the power of such a cultural change to impact values and operations. Investment bankers swoop down to push financing interests; public accounting firms add their flavor, while the public health and charitable goals of earlier generations fade. More and more business schools and health administration programs are training physicians to move ahead in the management of the field.

All of this consolidation leads to greater oligopoly and monopoly behavior. Unchecked, these developments could leave us with the worst of all worlds, namely, monopolistic pricing and a lack of community interest. There are two major counters to this trend: aggressive antitrust enforcement and aggressive buyer behavior that adds counterweights to large sellers. Since government is a big buyer, we are not without a potential public interest advocate with a stake in policing the industry. The health field will go through a long period of consolidation that will lead to more concentrated markets. When this happens it will be necessary for government to develop some form of utility regulation and control for the industry. On the positive side, many efforts are currently under way to try and find more efficient ways to deliver quality care. It is hard to imagine this happening without the kind of price pressures brought by managed care companies demanding discounts and more efficient delivery.

The old models of prepaid group practice and regionalization, while good ideas, never got off the ground. The possibility of obtaining some good, old-fashioned profits made the current business ventures attractive for investors, and it is having some payoff. Without a profit motive, change is not likely to occur. Assuming that the health field manages to avoid the monopoly trap of consolidation, whoever owns the industry in the future will have an integrated set of organizations. It is unlikely that there will be a countertrend toward the fragmentation that characterized the pre-1990s vertical integration movement.

Now that managed care is a firmly established trend, there is a high probability that more and more talent will enter the leadership ranks from among the leading members of medical disciplines. This infusion of talent can be expected to take managed care from its current price orientation to a more fundamental orientation of getting greater value for resources used.

Conclusions

A transformation of health care services is underway that is replacing a community and patient focus fueled by fee-for-service and cost-plus reimbursement with a focus on profit maximization. Managed care is shifting power away from professionals and communities into organizations financed by Wall Street. Even traditional community health care organizations are being driven by Wall Street, by using financial ratios as scoreboards to determine who gets the capital for growth and development.

Managed care is still generating high profits for HMOs, and money is being spent to increase market share through acquisitions, mergers, and new entries. As the market matures, price competition should begin to force HMOs to change. Physicians molded by high-quality patient-centered medical practice and further shaped by the mastery of management disciplines will be needed to run the vast systems required to tie everything together and finance it all.

The large risks and substantial dislocation that have resulted from managed care and the transformation of the health care field have led to an investor's world. The current course will eventually move to a higher plateau. Physicians will move in the direction of advanced managed care systems. This physician involvement will not, however, presage a return to the old ways of fee-for-service solo-practice medicine, or a move in the direction of government regulation.

Competition as a driving force and equity market financing have become the major winners. It will become increasingly necessary, however, to create greater values in care systems in order to keep the business. This will require a marriage among medicine, marketing, and general management. This marriage will be consummated by the management savvy of trained leaders from the ranks of specialty and generalist medicine. Health care reform will arise again through insurance reform, in response to problems of cost and access. The pressure to control cost will demand better methods, and a shift that will favor new leadership. There will be problems with this change, many unforeseen.

The times are changing, forcing organizations to change. Before we rest, more change will take place, making the health care field a continually challenging environment for a career.

Notes

1. This transition has been discussed in depth in a series of articles by Montague Brown and Richard Johnson. This chapter builds on that work. See *Health Care Management Review,* 1994, *19*(2, 3, 4); and *Health Care Management Review,* 1995, *20*(1, 2).
2. Anders, G. "Money Machines HMOs Pile up Billions in Cash, Try to Decide What to Do With It." *The Wall Street Journal,* December 21, 1994, p. 1.
3. Eckholm, E. "While Congress Remains Silent, Health Care Transforms Itself." *The New York Times,* December 18, 1994, p. 1.
4. Eckholm, E. "While Congress Remains Silent, Health Care Transforms Itself," p. 34.
5. Weil, T. P. "Close to a Bull's Eye: A Concurring Opinion." *Health Care Management Review,* 1995, *19*(2).
6. "AMA Shifts Focus to Incremental Reform." *American Medical Association News,* December 19, 1994, pp. 1, 24.
7. The first major book devoted to this trend was by Brown, M., and Lewis, H. L. *Hospital Management Systems: Multi-Unit Organization and Delivery of Health Care.* Germantown, Md.: Aspen Systems, 1976.
8. Miller, R. H., and Luft, H. S. "Managed Care Plan Performance Since 1980: A Literature Analysis." *Journal of the American Medical Association,* 1994, *271*(19), 1512–1519.
9. Miller and Luft, "Managed Care Plan Performance Since 1980."
10. For an in-depth treatment of opportunities for physicians in management see Brown, M. "Physician Opportunities in Management: Signs and Portents." *Physician Executive,* December 1994.

Chapter Eight

The Public's Future Perspective on Managed Care

Everett A. Johnson

Two respected long-term participants in health care administration are predicting managed care outcomes for a decade or so from now. Each participant has anticipated the same general direction for health care, but a somewhat different emphasis in outcomes.

One participant, Richard Johnson, believes that billion-dollar delivery systems operating integrated care programs on a for-profit basis will prevail. The other participant, Montague Brown, also foresees very large integrated systems operated on a nonprofit basis that will make major investments in prevention and wellness programs as a major part of their social mission. We may or may not wind up with integrated delivery systems that blend these projections in equity-based public utility companies that have major preventive health programs as essential elements of their cost-control strategy.

These forecasters have assumed that managed care programs will continue to grow because of their popularity with insurance carriers, employers, and government as the most effective way to moderate annual increases in health care expenditures. However,

Note: This chapter has been adapted from Johnson, E. "The Public's Future Perspective on Managed Care." *Health Care Management Review,* 1995, *20*(2). Copyright © 1996, Aspen Publishers, Inc. Used with permission.

the outcome they have not considered is the effect public opinion will have on determining the ultimate development of managed care strategies. What the American public expects from medical care services and how much they are willing to spend to support this system will determine the extent to which managed care becomes the primary vehicle for controlling medical care expenditures.

The current intense concern about the costs of medical care is the result of forty years or more of emphasis on the quality, availability, and range of medical services rather than on the expense of those services. This traditional priority has been stood on its head by managed care concepts that focus first on the costs of medical care. These programs see patients as cost centers to be controlled, rather than as people in pain, facing debilitating disease, or having anxiety attacks about their care.

Who Is in Charge?

The most fundamental question facing the health field in a managed care era is, Who is in charge: the patient, the physician, or the third-party payer? Managed care places medical care in a straitjacket. Patient choice is of less concern than reducing medical care expenditures. In the eyes of a third-party administrator, a cost-effective physician is more beloved than a caring physician who will order a marginally useful test to allay patient fears.

Since 1948, when the Wagner, Murray, Dingell bill to ensure health care through government intervention was proposed, the rallying cry of critics of government involvement in health care has been to prevent the enactment of socialized medicine. The essence of the opponents' argument has been that patients must be allowed the freedom to select their providers of care.

The Clinton administration's recent promotion of a federally controlled comprehensive health care plan attempted to mislead public opinion by saying that the plan offered free choice when in fact the legislation restricted physician choice. Many political analysts have expressed opinions that the 1994 mid-term election losses of the Clinton presidency were a response to this overly complex, too bureaucratic, impersonal health care legislation that was not supported by public opinion. Historically, Americans have preferred major social changes to occur gradually and piecemeal, rather than by a grand design.

The American body politic can be characterized as individualistic, self-determining, and resentful of limits on personal decision making. A fundamental strategy in managed care is to restrict patient choice of primary and specialist physicians and hospitals in order to control expenditures. It is worth noting that while this strategy is a step toward socializing medical care, it is promoted as procompetitive. However, when patients' choice of physician is restricted, managed care is not procompetitive for patients, only for insurers. As managed care savings decrease over time, it is likely that patient choice will progressively become more restricted, and onerous to the public.

The rapid growth of managed care in the private sector has not yet been recognized by broad public opinion because it does not have the visibility of government processes. As these plans expand, more and more people will become aware of their limitations, and public resistance to enrollment will gradually increase.

Cost reductions in health care expenditures are the outcome of reduced resource use; patient days, tests, fees, rates charged, convenience, employees, and so on can be eliminated or decreased in the delivery of medical care. The ultimate difficulty with managed care is that expenditure reductions are a one-time occurrence and are not repeatable. Once managed care savings are achieved, any future reductions must come through reduced illness and disease. Until morbidity is lowered, any increase in health care costs from inflation, new technology, or more resource use will result directly in increased health care insurance premiums.

As the payers of health care add restrictions that affect patients in order to offset cost increases, public acceptance and support of the managed care concept will wane, and eventually active opposition will develop. When this happens, physicians and hospital executives will support resistance and the patient's right to choose both physician and hospital providers.

The emerging milieu will be significantly different from the environment in which managed care became popular. The historical separation of physician from hospital will not recur. The effort to create health care systems that integrate medical practice and hospitals into one entity will not be disassembled. Gains in efficiency and coordinated care will not be discarded; rather, they will be the basis of the next evolutionary phase in medical care.

The public's reaction to the loss of personal control of their medical care will stimulate a new approach that will protect the patient's choice of physician and institutional care. In the past, insurance carriers struggled to find ways for patients to be cost conscious in their health care decisions. First, dollar coverage was modified by the use of coinsurance and deductible features. When these methods failed significantly to make patients aware of medical costs, the carriers instituted controls on patient choice by internal decision-making authorities that limited or prevented patient choice unless patients paid the total cost of their medical care. Second opinions, admission reviews, and utilization controls were initiated as managed care strategies, followed by the use of primary care physicians as gatekeepers and by capitation schemes, to provide insurance carriers with controls over patient decision making.

The implementation of these strategies has always been at cross-purposes with the desires of patients. The American public believes that medical care is a private matter that involves personal decisions and a confidential relationship with their physician. They believe that decisions about access to care and its quality and availability properly belong to patients and their physicians and should not be controlled by a remote, unidentifiable third party who is more concerned with costs than with care.

Competitive Programs

One way out of managed care control of patients and their involvement in economic decisions about medical care is the current effort by some carriers to bridge the gap between costs and patient choice with programs that include patient decision making. Whereas in managed care arrangements, bargaining occurs only periodically, when physician and hospital contracts are negotiated, in these competitive plans, physicians and hospitals are concerned daily with price and quality to avoid losing patients. While managed care programs focus on the organizational relationships among insurance carriers, physicians, and hospitals that structure the patient's interaction with the providers of care, competitive plans are keyed to individual patient expectations, needs, and choices. These competitive programs are based on individual patient decisions and thus create daily price and service demands on physicians and hospitals. They are in step with public demands for reduced government regulation.

Experienced health insurance carriers know that 5 percent of their policyholders will generate 90 percent of the costs of care, 45 percent of the policyholders will cause 10 percent of the expenditures, and 50 percent will incur no health care bills. This distribution of health care expenditures allows the carriers to identify and maintain weekly contact with patients who are actively using medical care services.

Assistance programs of this type are a return to patient choice, with knowledgeable patient agents representing the patient's financial interest to providers of medical care as they negotiate prices. They also allow a return to fee-for-service payments to physicians. This individualistic and competitive approach is personal and professional, and it replaces the bureaucratic rigidity of the impersonal managed care system. It is a sensible way to deal with price and market issues.

Conclusions

The 1994 election that overturned control of both houses in Congress is a harbinger of changes to come in health care. The American public has a fundamental belief that government policy and large, impersonal insurance carriers should not limit personal choice in the private matter of medical care. If the present mood of the American public prevails in managed care, as it has done in government regulation, a competitive system of health insurance based on patient choice should emerge as a major way to ensure health care.

The specter of major integrated organizations dominating a regional health care market will be moderated to some degree by the presence of competition. Competition for individual patients will impede the development of behemoth-sized integrated health care systems because large-scale medical care organizations lose economies of scale, as does large government.

As the financing of medical care evolves beyond managed care, the ultimate losers may be the large health insurance carriers. With integrated care systems at the local level, businesses that buy health insurance may decide to deal directly with the community health care system and eliminate the overhead costs of the insurance carrier.

The intrusion of managed care into the patient-physician relationship is unwelcome and often resented by patients and physicians. Once the cost savings have been gained, it is likely that public opinion will stimulate a return to patient choice in medical care. When public opinion coalesces against managed care, the eventual outcome may be overrated. The eventual outcome is unknown, but the current support for managed care plans will not last as patients increasingly sue these plans for inappropriate care.

Chapter Nine

Ethically Balancing Medical Care and Managed Care

Everett A. Johnson

Future opinions of managed care programs will ultimately hinge on the public's sense of how justly and fairly these programs are operated—and on how they affect people's relationships with physicians. Health care services are increasingly facing an ethical dilemma, as managed care in its many different shapes is often forcing physicians to choose between loyalty to patients and institutional policy. Divided loyalty has always existed at the outer edge of clinical decisions, where hard choices must be made, such as in the selection of a patient for a transplant. With the cost of medical care now a major economic concern, ethical dilemmas have become daily occurrences for physicians as they cope with managed care policies.

The promise of the Hippocratic oath, to keep patients free from harm and injustice, has traditionally guided physicians' motivations in medical care decisions. The primacy of the patient's welfare has been paramount and has required physicians to be free of any bias in order to take the right actions for each patient.

Ethical Dilemmas of Managed Care Practices

The managed care programs of the early 1970s foreshadowed the ethical choices that are now daily experiences for physicians and hospitals. The current popularity of managed care strategies is based on limited use of medical resources through judicious diagnostic and treatment decisions. Any gap between the concern for a patient's well-being and the reasonable use of resources is frequently an ethical dilemma for a physician, who must choose between loyalty to the patient and organizational priorities. Hospitals, likewise, create ethical dilemmas for themselves if they offer prices below the cost of the services provided when they bid for and enter into managed care contracts that discount their established rate structure. To offset the losses and to provide an operating margin, hospitals increase their rate structures to recover the discounted rates, as well as to generate a profit. By doing so, they disadvantage indemnity-insured and self-pay patients. Patients covered by managed care contracts have their hospital bills reduced by the percentage discounted, while other patients are billed at rates in excess of the costs of the services they receive. The latter rates provide an operating margin for the services provided to these patients, as well as making up for the loss of the operating margin of the managed care patients. This policy violates the economic principle that prices should be based on the costs of providing a service.

As the popularity of managed care programs has increased, some insurance carriers have further exploited patients financially. The more avaricious carriers have taken advantage of the coinsurance and deductible features of their policies by billing the managed care patients for the full amount of the difference from the established charges rather than according to the discounted rate structure. In the worst cases, the carriers then require hospitals to refund to them the difference between the full and discounted rates used to collect the coinsurance and deductible amounts. Each of these managed care practices have warped the traditional clinical, psychological, and financial concerns of ethical medical care delivery to a degree sufficient to place individual and institutional well-being ahead of the welfare of patients. Ethical dilemmas are inescapable in a relationship with a managed care program. As the number of people covered by managed care expands, there will also be an increase in the abuse of patients.

The managed care practice of denying claims for medical services provided by emergency rooms or for services outside the system and the practice of excluding particular physicians and hospitals from participation in a particular managed care program have forced patients to seek out new providers of care when joining a system. Both practices are at cross-purposes with patient welfare concerns.

The practices of managed care plans have shifted power from the patient-physician relationship to the managed care plan's outside interest, whose goal is maximization of profit. The result of this transfer of power is that the economic arrangements among physicians, hospitals, and insurance carriers are blurring the physician's responsibility for a clearly defined patient accountability.

The ethical responsibilities of a managed care organization are generally perceived to be the same as the customary duties and accountabilities of a business firm. Insurance carriers with managed care lines of business have applied their experience and the standards of the insurance industry to their health care programs. Their perspective is characterized by the use of the word "product" to describe the health insurance they provide, whereas medical care is characterized as a "service." There is a world of difference between products and services.

The Patient-Physician Relationship

The most fundamental characteristic of good quality medical care is trust between patients and physicians. However, the complexity of modern medicine often blinds patients to the dangers in the diagnosis and treatment modalities and the amount of harm a physician can cause patients. The bedrock of the healing process is a patient's trust in a physician's motivation to place the patient's well-being ahead of any other interest.

Managed care practices are an intrusion into a personal relationship that is recognized by law as private and confidential. To obtain health insurance coverage, policyholders are required to authorize release of their medical information to the carrier. During the era of first-dollar coverage, the availability of a patient's medical information was only rarely of significance. Current managed care practices now use patient information for commercial purposes that may compromise the honesty and ethics of patients, physicians, and hospitals. The dimensions of ethical abuse now reach in many directions and are often undetected.

The only purpose of medical care is the maintenance and restoration of the health of patients. That purpose is attenuated in managed care by the carrier's desire for profit maximization. In essence, business decisions override patient concerns. The carrier's approval or denial of a physician's clinical decisions directly affects patients.

Health care is moving into a new and strange era. In the past, it was believed essential that a physician's patient-centered decisions be unencumbered by organizationally imposed restraints. The decisions made in 1919 by the standardization program for hospital accreditation of the American College of Surgeons that established a separate medical staff for hospitals arose out of this concern. In the early years of the twentieth century, the government enacted licensing laws for physicians that aimed to protect patients, including laws preventing the corporate practice of medicine. The point was to protect medical care as an autonomous profession in order to maintain physicians' integrity in their patient-care relationships.

Control of Physician Decisions

In managed care programs, a physician's efforts may be constrained and thus at cross-purposes with the best care for patients. By denying payment of physicians' clinical orders, managed care programs compromise physicians' historical freedom of independent judgment. Denial of physicians' decisions ignores two important concerns: the practice of medicine is more experience and intuition than pure science, and the emotions of patients can be as upsetting as actual pain. High-quality patient care includes consideration of a patient's feelings when making diagnostic and treatment decisions. Physicians' concern for providing emotional support to patients comes from their experiences and insights, as they use their common sense to find practical ways to support a patient.

Implicit in a managed care strategy is a desire to restrain a physician's loyalty to patients through direct and indirect controls. Requiring physicians to get preadmission approval, meet utilization control criteria, follow diagnostic and treatment protocols, and refer only to approved specialists are the direct controls used to restrict physicians' decisions about patient care. Efforts to motivate physicians to conserve the use of patient care resources include the use of a capitated payment system, fee limitation, bonus payments, and economic credentialing reviews.

These types of incentives are two-edged swords. They encourage thoughtful use of patient care resources, yet they also motivate physicians to minimize diagnostic and treatment orders in order to earn additional income from incentive programs that reward reduced patient-care expenditures. The traditional fee-for-service payment system rewards physicians for increasing patient care services, but has led to abuse of patients through excessive diagnostic and treatment procedures.

Managed care strategies have also created hard choices for patients. The use of gatekeeper physician controls to prevent self-referral of patients to specialists, the use of utilization controls for admissions and length of stay, and the use of high-level deductibles and coinsurance for out-of-system medical services can be detrimental to patients.

Medical ethics do not require blind loyalty to patient-first criteria, no matter what the existing circumstances. Quality-of-life issues and extravagant use of resources to maintain life are important matters for a physician—and only for a physician. The practice of medicine requires the use of judgment. Society allows and protects a physician's freedom to make ultimate judgments about the care of patients where a reasonable certainty exists about outcomes. To alleviate the consequences of these ultimate-care decisions, physicians often share them with patients and family. As a profession, medicine has a responsibility that should not be compromised by managed care organizations.

Abuse of Patients

The difficulty, of course, is the variability of the knowledge and skill of individual physicians. Experience has shown that physicians have overtreated and overpriced, either through avarice or ignorance, or they have mistreated and undertreated patients. Whatever the abuse, the available remedies—medical staff reviews, credentialing, state licensure, malpractice lawsuits, and specialty certification—have limited but never abolished abuse of patients.

Conversely, the accountabilities of managed care organizations have been limited to insurance commissioner actions and lawsuits for contract violations. The opportunity to abuse patients is much broader when the ethics of business are the controlling criteria.

The standard of conduct in medicine is substantially higher than in business.

For hospitals, the imperatives of financial survival and success are distractions that may generate abuses to patients. The reimbursement methodologies of Medicare, Medicaid, and managed care have created a need for hospitals to adopt cost-shifting practices to maintain a financially stable operation. Hospitals have overcharged indemnity and self-pay patients in order to recover the deep discount losses from these programs. It is obvious that a policy of cost shifting is abusive to patients. Profit-maximizing behavior drives hospitals to serve those patients who pay the most.

The success of managed care programs in controlling rising medical care costs and in bringing about modest rate decreases has not benefited the purchasers of insurance coverage to nearly the same extent as the owners. Substantial profits have accrued without significantly lowering premiums, and resulted, as with hospitals, in taking advantage of the public.

The Future of Managed Care

The popularity of managed care concepts evolved from step-by-step rational economic decisions made in response to rapid price increases in medical care. These developments emphasized the achievement of short-term gains by price-shopping hospitals and medical services. They also stimulated the purchase of physician practices, the employment of physicians on a salary basis, and the creation of closed-panel referral networks to control primary care specialty referrals. The result of centralized planning has been tighter controls of medical care services. The strategy was to create greater uniformity and predictability in the volume of medical services by reducing the autonomy of stand-alone physician practices.

In a market economy, the collective opinion of the public will determine the acceptability of managed care. The ultimate test will be whether the public believes the policies of managed care will enhance or reduce the value of the medical services they receive. For example, managed care programs will control the acquisition of technology, but new innovations will sooner or later be demanded by the public. As medical technology continues to improve, it will lead to the identification of more disease. Until medical research can find ways to eliminate diseases, increases in the cost of medical services will be the direct result of increases in medical expenditures, once managed care savings are used up.

At its present stage of development, managed care has not been willing to come to grips with several key issues. The most obvious is a need to determine how funding for the education of medical personnel and support for medical research fit into the managed care paradigm. Another important issue is the role of managed care in community health programs that encourage immunizations, reduce teenage pregnancy, cope with the use of illegal drugs, and promote personal good health practices. Unless there are identifiable payoffs, managed care will not fund community health programs.

Because managed care organizations are becoming the primary way of funding health care programs, they should have the responsibility of supporting community health activities. Yet, despite statements made by many hospital associations and alliances that encourage local health care delivery systems to sponsor community health programs, economic reality will prevent serious efforts to do so, because hospitals and physician organizations are concerned with the pricing of their bids for medical service contracts and will exclude costs that cover optional program services. In the long run, leadership in this area will occur only when funding sources mandate and fund local activities. Both the insurance carrier and the health care delivery system have an ethical obligation to do so.

Abolishing Sacred Cows

For the past quarter of a century, the field of health administration has debated the desirability of and ethical justification for an investor-owned hospital system. Many not-for-profit hospital executives still believe that for-profit organizations are unethical and financially abusing patients. What is ignored is the abuse of patients and communities by not-for-profit hospitals that maintain excessive profit margins.

The fundamental issue is not profit versus nonprofit, or taxable versus tax-exempt status, but whether a hospital has demonstrated in its operating policies a concern for the welfare of the people in the community. From an ethical perspective, legal status is not a key criterion. Rather, it is availability and quality of care that demonstrates an organization's ethical standards of appropriate care. Ethically, both organizational forms are justifiable and should be judged by the degree to which they achieve the mission of providing medical care.

Another sacred cow is the belief that the consolidation of independent physician practices into large multispecialty group practices will improve the quality of care and the satisfaction of patients. The reality of group practice is somewhat different from this belief. In small, single-specialty group practices, patients expect to have a relationship with one physician, except for emergencies. Being treated by a partner of one's regular physician may be an unsettling experience. Different physicians have different personalities, which might cause a minor disturbance for a patient; but when the patient senses a significant difference, it is most likely that the physicians have different medical care values and philosophies.

Experience has shown that the process of selecting physicians for a group is most often limited to an evaluation of their skills, and little concern is shown for exploring their medical care philosophies. When large group practices are formed from the members of a hospital's medical staff, no effort is made to deal with the different values of individual physicians. Ignoring this issue will create unhappiness in these groups over time. In contrast, the Mayo Clinic physicians work at developing a unified perspective, and have been doing so for generations.

It is most likely that patient satisfaction and quality of care will decrease with the creation of large multispecialty group practices. It is also predictable that the physician with marginal skills who is also the least-expensive and most-modest user of medical resources will be able to hide behind the protective shield of a large group.

Another discontinuity in medical care is the policy of managed care organizations to avoid involvement in the provision of medical care while also insisting on controlling the utilization of medical services—the all or nothing approach to utilization decisions. The withholding of approval for a proposed expensive procedure is, for most patients, equivalent to denying treatment. In essence, interference with a physician's judgment is similar to practicing medicine when a barrier to the use of health services is present.

Denial of a request to approve a clinical procedure is an awkward process that leaves a trail of unhappy patients and physicians.

Conclusions

A person's individual attitudes are, in a sense, the application of their core moral beliefs that have been shaped by their earlier personal and professional experiences into judgments about ethical behavior. The commonly agreed upon ethical conduct for health care personnel is the promotion of the well-being of patients by the provision of quality care premised on a relationship of trust between patient and physician.

These ethical percepts have been compromised by managed care programs as they have developed strategies to decrease the rate of increase in medical care expenditures. Their utilization controls have been rationalized on the basis that the results justify the means used to reduce the rate of cost increases. Because health care is personal and centered on individuals, the goal of the greater good of society has no importance when medical care does not meet the needs of the individual.

To have a long-term future, managed care programs must recognize that ethical behavior is a two-way street and adopt policies that support trust between patients and physicians. The current rush to create huge managed care companies is driven by the market-oriented perspective that compromising the quality of care to increase profits and to somewhat decrease health insurance costs is an acceptable business practice, resulting in an acceptable trade-off.

A fundamental ethical concern is providing a sufficient financial basis for medical care and maintaining the freedom of patients to select their physicians. For physicians, the concern is to choose who they will serve. It is clear from experience that it is necessary to control the costs of medical care. It is likewise obvious that a significant percentage of patients and physicians have a sense that their interests are compromised by managed care policies.

Neither fee-for-service systems nor managed care have prevented ethical abuses in the delivery of medical care. On the one hand, fee-for-service has encouraged cost increases that affect the availability of medical care for the larger community; on the other hand, managed care has discouraged medical care for individuals. To unwittingly take advantage of the system is excusable, but to deliberately abuse the system is unethical.

To achieve an ethically balanced method of paying for medical services, the needs of patients must be met while improving control of the costs of medical care. To do so requires that both the providers and financiers of medical care be accountable for their decisions. Because of the intertwining and complexity of required judgments, no system that serves both interests will achieve perfection, but there is a need to create a definitive accountability of providers for the quality of care and of managed care organizations for the financing of medical care.

The accountability of physicians and hospitals for maintaining an acceptable standard of care has steadily expanded in this century, from licensing, increasing malpractice exposure, accreditation, and board certification, to medical staff credentialing and reappointment reviews. The most pervasive accountability has been the national accreditation program for hospitals that also affects physician performance. Since the program's establishment in 1919, accreditation criteria have been progressively improved and refined, and they are once again undergoing a major reorganization to improve their effectiveness.

Although insurance carriers are licensed, their accountability is more limited than that of hospitals and centers on the carriers' capacity to have sufficient funds available to pay claims. Their operational standards are enforceable at the state level and are generically rather than specifically related to health care services. The result of these standards is that accountability is not evenly balanced between the providers of care and those who pay for it. The effort to cope with differing levels of ethical conduct suggests that some type of external criteria need to be used to evaluate performance and maintain ethical behavior. The accomplishments of the voluntary accreditation program for hospitals and its effect on physician behavior suggest that, even though the program was not totally successful, a similar broad-scope accreditation program for accrediting managed care programs would accomplish a similar upgrading and reinforcement of ethical behavior. While there are now accreditation programs in operation that have evaluation criteria for managed care programs, there is a need to establish standards that integrate both outcomes and internal operations; that evaluate relationships with patients, physicians, and hospitals; and that measure a wide range of factors. The key to establishing broader and deeper managed care standards would be to allow their application to be reflected by variations in an operating philosophy rather than to be judged according to precise criteria that preclude modifications that would take place with longer experience.

The establishment of a voluntary accreditation program with a depth and breadth of evaluating criteria would probably deter efforts to enact a federally sponsored program for managed care programs. If managed care is to have a long-term future, the public must be satisfied that their medical care is not compromised by the arbitrary decisions of carriers.

It will never be easy to define standards of conduct for managed care organizations that equally balance community good with the well-being of the individual. However, over time and through experience, an organized, voluntary, broad-ranging accreditation program will have a better chance of approaching that goal than federally enacted controls of managed care.

Chapter Ten

A Personal Encounter with Managed Care

Montague Brown

America's so-called health care system has a lot of gaps, many of which are downright dangerous to a person's health. If a physician can correctly diagnose and treat a problem without outside help and referrals, the "system" works well. But if one must depend on the system to refer one to the proper place for the proper diagnosis and treatment, the continuity factor falters badly, and in the much-touted managed care organization things may be even worse than in the traditional system. The result: less quality at greater cost.

Things are going from bad to worst! As a concept, health maintenance seems sound enough. Its proponents, often including me, seem sincere in wanting to keep folks healthy. But well-meaning people doing their best is just not good enough. Managed care seeks low-priced, low-cost care in order to achieve maximum profits to "managers," providers, and others. Promoting the idea of health maintenance or prevention may be good marketing, but as a norm for practice, it is pure myth. Consumers can and often do end up with more-expensive and lower-quality care, and unfortunately, in this respect both for-profit and not-for-profit managed care systems look very much alike.

Note: This chapter has been adapted from Brown, M. "A Patient Encounter with Managed Care: A Painful Experience." *Health Care Management Review,* 1990, *15*(4), 5. Copyright © 1990, Aspen Publishers, Inc. Used with permission.

How can one come to such a radical conclusion without tons of research, years of careful studies, and panel after panel of experts to judge quality? It is simple: try the system for yourself. Ray Brown, the most astute observer of health care in this century, often remarked that quality would become more problematic once providers earned more while spending less time and resources on serving clients. Frankly, health care is experiencing many problems outside of prepaid, managed care systems, but managed care adds its own negative twist to the system failure being experienced today.

My own trial of the system occurred recently. "A stress-fractured femur," said the doctor. Because of the possibility of slippage of the fracture, hip joint replacement might be required—if the bone is not pinned (nailed, actually) to secure it for proper healing. This type of fracture shows up poorly on X-rays; a bone scan is required for proper diagnosis.

Knowing of my HMO's propensity for anticipating self-healing (take an analgesic and wait two weeks), at the onset of pain I treated myself. After two weeks, a primary care physician took an X-ray and prescribed the same course of treatment I had just undergone.

After the primary physician's enforced two additional weeks of waiting failed to produce improvement, another week was lost getting a referral to an orthopedic specialist at a teaching hospital. As an HMO patient, I had the honor of being teaching material for a resident, who appeared to be on his first stint in the clinic. What did this team do? They chose to start at square one. A different analgesic, a month-long wait, and then, "If the pain persists, you can have the bone scan, provided the HMO authorizes the follow-up."

The HMO and referring physician ignored the patient. The referring physician ignored both the patient and the primary care physician's treatment. This failure to listen, counsel, and act on what others had found cost the patient pain and work loss, and risked unnecessary complications. Smart medicine? No. Cheap medicine? No. Quality medicine? No. More expensive and poorer quality medicine at higher cost to the consumer.

A colleague who is a veteran of years of study of the U.S. medical care system remarked that my experience represents the more typical encounter with managed care. A recent health problem in his family brought different horror stories, but a similar conclusion: consumers of managed care plans run great personal risk of getting poor quality care at high cost. Worse still, the danger only gets seen when the client is already in the system, with no options for getting out, except at very high cost.

Many good people helped me in this encounter. Clerks smiled and apologized for the lack of data integration that forces the ill to undergo multiple inquiries needlessly. The physical therapist was nice, but could offer no advice on rehabilitation since no doctor's orders on it were available. The surgeon ultimately did an excellent job, or so it seems. He did tear a bit of flesh when the staple extractor was turned upside down mistakenly, and he allowed that almost any exercise was good if no weight was on the leg. The HMO protocol pushers stick to their guns: in the face of client threats to leave the system, they insist that you cannot take the X-ray with you!

Properly implemented, this system could have produced good quality at reasonable cost to both the provider and the consumer. But well-meaning, good people failed to deliver quality care at reasonable cost. Unfortunately, the primary mission of almost everyone I encountered during this sorry episode seemed to be protecting their immediate turf, treating the consumer in the narrowest manner possible. The cutting, nailing, sewing, and stapling works well. Connections with different levels of care, across professional lines, and between professionals and clients failed.

Managed care fails in many ways. Neither prevention nor first-rate specialist care exists—only strictly rationed medical services. Primary physicians in managed care plans seem locked to protocols that detract from their ability to treat patients as individuals. The sense of a system of connectedness seems nonexistent. Rationing patterns and methods alienate contracting physicians and other providers, adding to the poisoning of their relationships with clients. The cost of management systems lowers the value delivered to consumers, while raising the cost of what is provided in service.

Can these flaws be cured? Perhaps, but not without recognition by physicians, managers, insurers, business, government, and more importantly, consumers that our system of medical care is sick. It is not self-correcting. It cannot be designed from the outside, nor do those on the inside appear to have the courage to face up to its most grievous ills. Medical care organizations are tough to change. Almost anyone can veto change, and few changes can be made without appearing to threaten someone.

Managed care keeps moving along, but in practice it offers no pat solution to quality, cost, comprehensiveness, continuity, and access. Consider it another slick marketing device to extract consumer dollars. When this approach fails, more and fancier schemes will follow. Count on it.

One change must occur. Consumers must be listened to as whole people and not as discrete medical specialty areas. Physicians must listen to one another. It is unforgivable in any system of medical care for physicians and health professionals to lose the essential quality of the profession: the client is and must remain the primary beneficiary of all professional service. Forget that and we are doomed. Today, this essential underpinning of professionalism is at great risk. Retrieve it and the profession, the system, the individual client, and the public will benefit.

Note

1. Editorial. *Health Care Management Review,* 1990, *15*(2).

Hospital Governance in New Roles

Chapter Eleven

The Purpose of Hospital Governance

Richard L. Johnson

The purpose of hospital governance is defined by state statute, but how hospital governance carries out its responsibilities and defines its role is in the process of change. Historically, the hospital has been the centerpiece of a loosely coordinated delivery system held together primarily by informal relationships. As organized delivery systems, payer organizations, and physician groups develop contractual and corporate structures, the hospital is most likely to be replaced by one of them. Should this occur, the transition will be made painfully and unwillingly, as long-standing customs and traditions of hospital governance give way to a new order in which the hospital no longer dominates the health care scene.

The Changing Role of Governance

With change now sweeping the health care field, the community hospital is caught up in the tide, along with physicians and other health care providers. The focus of change is on managed care and the ways in which it will bring about new organizational and corporate structures among providers. Hospitals are seeking network

Note: This chapter has been adapted from Johnson, R. L. "The Purpose of Hospital Governance." *Health Care Management Review,* 1994, *19*(2), 81–88. Copyright © 1994, Aspen Publishers, Inc. Used with permission.

partners, developing physician-hospital organizations, management services organizations, and organized delivery systems, in an effort to keep the role of the hospital intact. In the course of all the organizational maneuvering that is going on, little attention is being devoted to examining the traditional organizational structure of the hospital to determine if it can meet the challenges now confronting it.

Years ago, in writing "The Three-Legged Stool,"[1] I indicated my concern that the typical structure of board-administration-medical staff was one that probably could not stand under a great deal of external pressure, such as is now being experienced. It is clear that these structures will be modified, altered, or radically changed in response to the new economic environment that is developing. Given these new external factors, it seems to be an appropriate time to ask a fundamental organizational question: What is the purpose of hospital governance?

Is it, as it has been throughout the twentieth century, to establish policy? To control, to plan, and to approve the activities of the hospital? Is it to see that the best possible care is provided at the lowest possible price, or to represent the community's health needs and see to it that the hospital is responsive to these concerns? Do these definitions satisfy the extent of the emerging role of the hospital?

Looked at from the reverse direction, the question might be, What is lost if a hospital has no governing board? Since approximately one-third of all hospitals in the United States do not have governing boards, how are their roles different from those that do have governing boards? The for-profit chains have corporate boards, but only advisory bodies at each participating institution. The military, Veterans Administration, and other federal hospitals have no governing boards, and some hospitals operated by cities or counties do not have boards. As managed care organizations grow and operate their own hospitals, they are most likely to centralize decision making at the corporate level, following the pattern of the for-profit hospital chains.

What is it that gives a hospital governing board its legitimate role? It could be argued that it is the state law defining the basic elements of a corporation, requiring corporate officers and a governance function. Yet, in and of itself this is a weak reed upon which to define a real role for governance. When stripped to the bare essentials, there can only be one purpose that sustains any action of a corporation, be it a hospital or any other form of enterprise: the governing board, through its collective decisions, *adds value* to the functioning of the organization. If value is not added, the board serves no useful organizational purpose, even though it may provide satisfaction to the individual members of that body, or satisfy state law.

What constitutes added value has changed over the decades. From the turn of the century through the 1950s, a governing board's added value was its ability to contribute money, either for capital or to cover operating losses at the end of each year. Hospitals were charitable institutions and philanthropy played an important role. Following World War II, a technological explosion dramatically increased the comprehensiveness of services provided in hospitals. Hospitals no longer depended on charitable contributions, but instead were reimbursed by third-party payers for their costs of operation. Increasingly, hospitals came to balance their social commitment with a business-like approach to earning revenues.

By the last decade of this century, hospitals had been transformed into technological enterprises dominated by business and professional expertise. Philanthropy was no longer of major interest, and the social responsibilities of serving the health needs of the community had become tightly controlled. In a very real sense, hospitals had become big business, often the largest or one of the largest employers in town. In terms of the nation's economy, health care came to account for one-seventh of all expenditures of the gross domestic product.

In light of this radical societal change in the role of the hospital, it is now relevant to ask about the purpose of hospital governance and its role in the coming years as new paradigms take root. As the health field shifts its focus to coping with managed care and the movement of large blocs of patient contracts from one hospital to another (depending upon how successful in bidding one provider is over another), the role of the governing board will once again undergo a change. As the percentage of managed care patient days continues to grow and as it combines with the percentage of Medicare days and approaches four-fifths or more of total patient days, the boards will require members with new and different talents, skills, and backgrounds. To successfully negotiate with managed care plans, business coalitions, or self-funded corporations, physicians and hospitals will have to bid jointly for their business. Whether the bidding body is a physician/hospital organization (PHO) or some other, similar organizational mechanism, the role of the hospital will no longer be central. Hospital governance will primarily deal with the problem of containing costs in order to be priced competitively. In an economic climate in which the goal is not revenue generation but control of expenses, the skills needed are managerial, financial, and operational.

The Shift to Managed Care

As coping with managed care becomes the dominant concern of hospitals, the skills represented on existing governing boards need to be reconsidered. The ability to forge strong physician-hospital relationships will be an essential ingredient. Basic to these relationships will be the ability of hospitals and physicians to mesh clinical and economic decision making with operational support from hospital personnel under restricted budgets. As revenues for both hospitals and physicians become more constrained, it will be more difficult to keep the physician-hospital relationship positive. The greater the in-depth knowledge that exists around the hospital governing board table, the more likely it will be that these difficulties can be ironed out.

Premium judgment will be focused on balancing the clinical needs of patients with the economic realities that must be considered in providing for their care. This judgment will require a combination of physicians and senior management. Inevitably, the traditional role of the governing board as conservators or trustees will be reduced. The value added to the functioning of the organization will occur at the senior management level. Being able to determine the amount of risk required to successfully bid for managed care contracts is a judgment call based on operational and clinical expertise. If revenues remain at the same level while inflation continues, the value added to the organization will come from the management of the operations, not from the board.

Further complicating the situation is the shift to ambulatory services as a result of advances in medical technology that require a meshing of outpatient and inpatient services. A growing number of clinical procedures are now performed on an ambulatory basis. Many procedures that do not require major capital expenditures will be shifted to physicians' offices if they can be safely performed in that setting. Decisions about which procedures can be shifted are made not by hospitals but by practicing physicians, independent of a hospital's wishes. While physicians are adding value to their practices by adding outpatient procedures, there is a loss of value to the hospital. The role of the governing board is to understand that this loss cannot be avoided, and then to plan for innovative joint activities with physicians. The development of management services organizations provides the opportunity to limit loss of revenue by creating new services that supplement the activities of physicians' practices. Developing such opportunities is a management responsibility, and once the concept has been approved by the board, the governance function is no longer involved.

A Collective Authority

Since a governing board is composed of a number of individuals, its authority is collective. The group meets together, discusses issues, and arrives at a consensus about a course of action or new policy that they all believe will add value. Experienced board members recognize that a collective decision requires consensus, so it is fundamentally important that the individual members share a common understanding about their roles and the direction of the organization. Collective decisions enable the hospital to follow a steady, thoughtful course and not constantly change direction, which confuses stakeholders and leads to a lack of support. A simple majority vote is not enough of a basis for proceeding on a course of action. Such a decision indicates substantial disagreement among board members. A wiser course of action is to delay or table the action. The belief that it is important to maintain a board size of an odd number in order to avoid ties is not an important consideration. A plurality of one is not a substantial agreement.

A board must have substantial agreement on decisions if those decisions are to be effectively implemented. Since a board is composed of individuals who are equal in terms of voting rights, it follows that all members are equally responsible for the decisions reached. Therefore, each member is equally entitled to participate in the discussions and votes. Such matters cannot be left to a selected few board members; board members who do not participate abrogate their responsibilities.

The development of governing board executive committees that tend to make all, or nearly all, of the governing board's decisions represents an abuse of authority. As often defined in the bylaws of a hospital corporation, executive committees are created to cope with urgent matters that cannot be delayed until the entire board can be assembled. Even when the members of the executive committee are the officers of the corporation, they must have their actions ratified at the next regularly scheduled board meeting.

The abuse of executive committee functioning occurs when the committee routinely considers matters that are not urgent and reaches decisions that properly belong on the agenda of the governing board. The use of an executive committee to act on all or most matters prior to submission to the full board is most often justified on the basis that the officers are the most knowledgeable and experienced persons associated with the hospital. Viewed from the perspective of value added, one of two conclusions can be drawn. On the one hand, if the decisions of the executive committee do in fact add value, then to permit their decisions to go before the full board takes away value if the full board does anything beyond being a rubber stamp. Under such circumstances, the governing board should be reduced to the size of the executive committee. Board members should be unwilling to serve where they are not accorded equal rights as board members, since they are regarded as providing less value to the organization than the value provided by executive committee members. On the other hand, if the full board adds value to the work of the organization, then it must insist that the organization is not receiving full value by relying so heavily on the executive committee, because board members are being denied the opportunity to participate in the governance function.

It is important for all board members to have a common commitment to the success of the institution and to accept the primacy of the institution in establishing policies. If board members believe that they represent the community to the hospital, they deny the primacy of the institution's goals and replace them with other goals. This does not mean that the hospital should be unconcerned about the community's interests, but rather that the hospital selects health goals from among the health needs of the community and decides which ones to serve. Since community interests are wider and broader than those of a hospital, it is necessary for the institution's goals to be within that scope, unless the governing board elects to adopt a different value system, as did the Mayo Foundation, the Cleveland Clinic, the Columbia Health System, or Kaiser-Permanente. If governance is to add value to the functioning of the organization, it must respond by providing policies that are aimed at perpetuating the hospital, not at perpetuating the community. That is someone else's job. The process of selecting institutional goals and the decisions reached by the governing board are what add value to the institution.

Since the primary responsibility of the hospital's board is to perpetuate the institution's existence (if the hospital is to serve the selected health needs of the community, the hospital must continue to exist), the focus of the governing board must be on long-term planning, and it must deal primarily with strategic issues rather than with operational matters.

Put in simple terms, operational matters are the province of the hospital's senior management, who are much more familiar with these matters than the members of the governing board. The board's interest in operational matters should be limited to an oversight function that answers the question, Are the long-term objectives of the hospital being jeopardized by any of the operational activities? Once this question has been answered, the focus of the board should shift back to its primary concern—the long-term strategic issues—where its greatest value can be found.

Added value also requires stability and continuity of leadership of the organization. If board members or the chief executive officer are replaced too frequently, the goals and plans of the organization will be in flux, which will result in a loss of value through a constant reordering of priorities. Projects will be started and aborted before being completed, or if completed, before full value can be achieved.

Measuring the Governance Function

Adding value to the functioning of a hospital is the responsibility of both the individual board members and the board as a whole. When individual board members have their own agendas that are separate from the common good, value is lost rather than added. If, for example, a board member views every issue on the agenda for its impact on a personal cause that has overriding importance for that board member—such as environmental concerns—there is a loss of value to the hospital organization.

If added value is the way to measure the worth of the governance function, then each board member's contribution to added value needs to be evaluated periodically and an overall judgment needs to be made. This process requires more than each member's evaluation of his or her own contributions. People with an intimate knowledge of the workings of the governing board need to be involved in deciding individual value added. Value is not determined by how many board meetings were attended; rather, the criteria have to reflect the individual's contribution to the shaping of the decisions collectively adopted by the board.

Two possible methods exist for making evaluations of the individual board members. The most logical approach is for the nominating committee to undertake this task. Since bylaws typically charge this committee with both recommending new members and reviewing reappointment of incumbents, an annual examination of the performance of existing board members can provide the basis for a committee's recommendations. To clarify its role as part of governance, the nominating committee might properly be renamed the nominating and evaluating committee.

In nonprofit organizations such as community hospitals, it is difficult to get committee members to accept the responsibility for annually evaluating the performance of each member of the governing board. Since board positions are typically unpaid, there is a reluctance to subject members to evaluation. However, if evaluation does not take place there is no uniform way of measuring individual performance to determine if he or she is adding value to the functioning of the organization. Because of the social nature of the nonprofit board, it is assumed that giving of one's time is the equivalent of adding value—a false assumption.

If having a nominating and evaluating committee is not acceptable, then the members of the governing board may wish to evaluate each other, acting as a committee of the whole. Each board member evaluates all other board members, but not his or her own performance. The nominating and evaluating committee, or the officers of the corporation, aggregate all of the scores on each individual board member, divide the total by the number of those voting, and obtain a score. By having a predetermined acceptable minimum score, it is possible to determine which board members are not adding value to the board's decisions in the eyes of the other board members. (See Table 13.2 in Chapter Thirteen for a list of actions that board members commonly perceive as adding or subtracting value.)

Credentialing Physicians

One of the major activities of the hospital governing board has been the review and approval of the process of credentialing the medical staff. The board grants the privileges, and the extent of them, for individual physicians to practice in the hospital. As a result of the development of organized delivery systems (ODSs), the value of having the governing board credential physicians has substantially decreased because one of the ODS's major functions is economic and clinical credentialing of its participating physicians. To be effective in securing managed care contracts, the ODS must concern itself with both clinical competence and economical practice patterns. Credentialing must still be accomplished by the hospital governing board for those physicians who have medical staff privileges but who, for whatever reason, are not participating physicians in the ODS. While the participating physicians in the ODS may be one-half or less of the total membership of the medical staff, they are likely to be the most active users of the hospital. The ODS physicians may account for 90 to 95 percent of hospital revenue.

As hospital revenues become more and more restricted, and in order to replace value lost by the governing board as ODS and managed care have grown in importance, philanthropy may be reinstituted as a board activity. This is unlikely, however, to become a major activity, and it certainly will not have the degree of importance it had prior to World War II. Over the intervening years, hospitals have moved further and further away from a charitable, social role and have become technological enterprises. In the process, the size of hospitals and the scope of their services have grown, and they have relied more and more on payment for services rendered.

If the history of American business can be used as a guide for hospitals, the freestanding, independent institution—the "mom and pop" operation—will be replaced by sophisticated, in-depth management that controls large blocs of health care resources at multiple locations. In such a setting the governing board is most likely to be concerned with long-term capital needs and an in-depth understanding of debt markets. As the health care corporation becomes a mixture of nonprofit and for-profit corporations, the board will have to be knowledgeable of equity markets as well. It may on occasion have a for-profit subsidiary that has such potential that it may be prudent to list shares of the subsidiary corporation on a stock exchange and be publicly traded. If this trend should develop over the next decade or two, hospital governing boards will closely resemble the governing boards of large business corporations.

Networks and Mergers

The odds are good that, as an inevitable result of managed care, the listing of shares on the stock market will become reality. There is a growing recognition among hospital chief executives that the independent, freestanding community hospital appears to have a limited future, unless it joins a network of hospitals or consolidates or merges with other hospitals. The reasoning behind this movement is that a lone hospital is not of sufficient size or economic strength to become a major player in a managed care environment. When the purchasers of health care services control vast resources with great economic strength, they can leverage any local market. Hospitals see it as necessary to band together to offset this advantage.

The scramble to form hospital networks is fundamentally based on the concept that if several hospitals form an economic bloc, the chances of survival are enhanced for all of those who join. The desire to survive is in keeping with the governing board's responsibility for assuring perpetuation of the hospital and does not jeopardize the autonomy of the participants. This course of action is, from a board perspective, adding value to the hospital. In deciding on this course of action, the board is assuming that a continuation of the hospital is needed by the community in which it is located. The fact that the community may be overbedded, and may become even more overbedded in the coming years, is not equal in importance to the board's responsibility to assure perpetuation of the institution. Rather than face the issue of closing the hospital, governing boards are most likely to seek network affiliations. Closing a hospital represents failure and a total loss of value to a governing board, while joining a network is thought of as adding value.

Mergers and consolidations of hospitals are readily understandable when looked at from the perspective of value added or value lost. When the merger is between for-profit hospitals, both parties are left with something of value. The surviving hospital anticipates adding value by having an additional facility at its disposal. The other hospital receives value through the dollars paid for the transfer of assets and liabilities. Both boards conclude that they have added value. However, when two hospitals that are nonprofit or public corporations merge and only one corporation survives, the values are different. The surviving hospital board has added value. The other hospital board has, in its own way of thinking, failed and lost value. Board members who serve the "failed" hospital will cling to the notion that they have protected the community's health needs by merging, but they are acutely aware that as a board they have failed to assure the perpetuation of the hospital corporation and there has been no exchange of value in return for the decision reached. For-profit hospitals do not have to be failing financially in order to merge, because there is an exchange of value. Nonprofit or public hospitals that merged into surviving institutions typically are in or near financial distress before facing up to reality. Board members of such hospitals find it difficult to make a decision to merge when the only outcome is a loss of value.

Conversely, when consolidation is explored by hospital governing boards—when two existing corporate structures are abandoned and a new third corporation is formed that acquires the assets and liabilities of the two original corporations—the answer to the question of adding or losing value is different. In consolidation, the basis of the effort is that the board members of both hospitals enter into negotiations believing that a favorable decision adds value. One does not gain while the other loses; rather, the consolidation is viewed as a win-win situation. When consolidation is not achieved but is terminated prior to the final vote, the issues that prevent consolidation involve other factors such as religious sponsorship, selection of a chief executive, or medical staff perceptions about how consolidation might affect their practices.

New Opportunities and Threats

Since the two driving forces of a hospital governing board are to add value to the functioning of the organization and to perpetuate the hospital's existence, the question of how these two forces will play out in the changing health care environment is of interest. An estimate of the changes likely to take place provides an avenue for understanding how hospital governing boards may be affected.

The health care environment is now undergoing drastic revisions, creating both new opportunities and new threats. From the viewpoint of the hospital, the economic climate is becoming much more risky. As the number of persons covered by managed care contracts grows and as the debate over setting a national number for total annual health care expenditures becomes an issue, the quest for continual improvement in hospital productivity stresses the importance of management in bringing about the needed results. In the matters of enhancing efficiency and securing managed care contracts the hospital governing board becomes a bystander, neither adding nor subtracting value to the functioning of the institution. Getting board members to accept the role of bystanders may be difficult. As unpaid volunteers dedicated to the matters of health care they may continue to view their roles as community representatives in an environment that has become increasingly competitive. In a hostile setting where there are both winners and losers, where community values do not prevail, and where the philosophical underpinnings of the board's values are in flux but headed toward becoming much more entrepreneurial, the problem that must be faced is determining what board decisions will add value to the hospital in an intensely competitive environment. Individual evaluations must take into account deciding that risk taking and entrepreneurial values are of primary importance.

The composition of the board needs to be examined. The sets of unique skills required to deal effectively with a managed care environment need to be determined and persons identified who can bring this type of knowledge to the boardroom. At the same time, those board members need to be identified who lack the aptitude, temperament, and knowledge to add value to board decisions in the emerging environment.

Given a choice, hospital board members and chief executives would probably choose a health care climate that fosters cooperation and coordination among providers and a friendly "we will work together" relationship with the payers. Realistically, this will not happen. The payers have determined that the day of "provider dominance" is over and it is now time to force a competitive mode of doing business on both physician and hospital providers. The climate this will create will be one of cost cutting, loss of income for both physicians and hospital employees, and an overriding concern with organizational survival. Hospital employees will fear the loss of their jobs, needed capital expenditures will be deferred, clinical programs that lose money will be terminated, and resentment among board members toward other hospitals and newly formed health care provider organizations will grow. As a result, board discussions and decisions are apt to focus on reacting to events and to pay insufficient attention to positive long-range planning for the future of the hospital.

As revenues become more and more limited, the role of the governing board will become less and less relevant because the kinds of decisions needed will be operational rather than strategic. Over the next few years, the governing board agenda will be concerned with the working out of formal structures for organizational relationships with physicians and other health providers, and perhaps with developing captive purchasers of services. Governing boards will have to make harsh, tough decisions that are unavoidable if they are to continue to add value. Making the right decisions for the right reasons will increasingly require board members who can function in the face of adversity. The sign that stood on

President Truman's desk when he was in the White House aptly describes the type of board member that will be needed: "If you can't stand the heat, get out of the kitchen." In the days that lie ahead, governing boards that add value are likely to have to be tough, fair-minded persons who are unconcerned about winning popularity contests. Sitting on a hospital governing board that will have to handle the rough and tumble of intense competition will be no place for the faint-hearted. Making sure that the board adds value to the functioning of the hospital will be a demanding task that will need to be approached through individual, annual evaluations of board member performance in order to assure that the collective decisions reached are appropriate to assuring the perpetuation of the hospital. In addition, the governing board will need to determine how its role will change in relationship to the role of senior management, carefully assessing the circumstances under which it will add value to the functioning of the hospital. Having made this determination, an inventory of needed skills, talents, and experiences will be required if the composition of the board is to fit the external environment in which the hospital must function.

Community Networks

The need to relate the hospital to what is happening in the external environment has led to a widespread opinion among hospital board members that joining a community network is a satisfactory alternative to merger or consolidation with other local hospitals. By limiting the hospital's participation to cooperation, the governing board maintains total control. Under this circumstance, the network must depend on the goodwill of the participating hospitals to accomplish its objectives. As a result, networks are weak organizational structures that lack the authority to require compliance with their programmatic decisions. Even though hospitals are driven to join networks by the fear of future economic consequences, boards and CEOs are reluctant to cede any real authority to another organization because that would represent a loss of control.

Loss of control is a primary concern until a hospital is directly faced with a disastrous financial condition; then merger or consolidation may be possible. Since networks can be joined without a loss of autonomy, they are viewed favorably as a way of coping with the threats posed by managed care organizations. At the same time, joining a network demonstrates that a hospital is primarily interested in entering into affiliations that are cooperative rather than competitive. Board members and CEOs are well aware that intense competition between local hospitals is costly to the community without offsetting value, because hospital competition is programmatic rather than economic. Duplicate services are costly. For example, two hospitals may each have an open heart program, but neither operates at full capacity.

The reasons for not going further and agreeing to consolidation or merger are noneconomic and typically lie below the surface of overt board concerns. Consolidations and mergers will be slow in coming as governing boards invoke real or imagined concerns with religious differences, public versus nonprofit status, unequal financial resources, or the desire of medical staffs to play off one hospital against another. Until managed care is able to control large blocks of patients, hospitals will most likely maintain their independence.

Hospital leadership is generally supportive of eliminating wasteful duplication of facilities and services among local hospitals, but when faced with the reality of potentially losing patient revenues because the neighboring hospital commences a new service or begins buying physician practices, the urge to compete takes over. The network or affiliated organization is helpless in preventing this competition because it has no authority. The governing boards of both competing hospitals may have serious reservations about what is going on, but they may also believe that their primary responsibility as board members is to add value to their own hospital, so they agree to decisions that heighten competition. Local coordination and cooperation disappear when only one hospital in a community elects to play the competitive game.

Conclusions

Competition between local hospitals can be expected to continue unabated and will grow in intensity proportional to the growth of managed care in the community. Hospital leadership will continue to give lip service to concerns about the community good, but community good will run a poor second in importance when hospital boards are faced with stiff competition from other hospitals. In the final analysis, board members understand that their role adds value when concerned with the perpetuation of the organization and loses value when the role of the hospital is compromised. Board members will reluctantly accept the necessity for their hospital to participate in the growing competition between institutions; they will not like it, but they will be unable to avoid it if they are to continue to add value in their collective role.

Note

1. Johnson, R. L. "The Three-Legged Stool, Part I." *Osteopathic Hospitals,* 1977, *21*(6), 14–16; Johnson, R. L. "The Three-Legged Stool, Part II." *Osteopathic Hospitals,* 1977, *21*(7), 12–15.

Chapter Twelve

Commentary
The Purpose of Hospital Governance Is . . . Purpose!

Montague Brown

The current health care environment presents a variety of challenges to hospital governance. One need not worry about trustees getting caught up in operations, provided that administration puts the real governance agenda on the table. I suggest several issues for starters:

1. Is a hospital of this type essential to supplying medical services in light of the various trends in managed care, ambulatory technology, and reform? If not, to what purpose might the assets we control be better utilized?
2. If one considered what a comprehensive integrated service might look like under various managed care and reform scenarios, how might our assets best be deployed to play an effective role?
3. Given the population base required to support a full-service system, do we currently serve a sufficient base to aspire to lead

or be a part of such a system? If not, with whom might we need to join to establish such a system?

4. Given the possible alternative system configurations that might best serve the medical care needs of this and adjacent communities, which ones seem most likely to succeed, and how might we go about testing the waters on developing such a system?

5. Do we have the requisite knowledge, sensibilities, and leadership to ask the right questions and to gather information to properly reflect on these issues?

These are the kinds of questions that need to be at the top of any agenda that deals with effectiveness of trustees and governance. All of these questions deal with fundamental purpose, a core trustee issue.

Richard Johnson has stimulated my thinking, as he often does, about this subject. But his approach in Chapter Eleven leaves me with a sinking feeling that he is on the wrong track—a feeling that goes against my knowledge of his work and ideas. Is his portrayal of governance in the industry correct? I fear that it is, because the opinion of health care executives is that the role of trustees should be that narrow role of supporting the existing institutional configuration and deploying assets. Constituencies array themselves around such totem poles. Governance must ultimately and continuously judge whether the purpose of governance needs to be changed in order to successfully capture opportunities for optimum asset deployment for the future. Administrators and physicians are the primary beneficiaries of a model of governance that says that trustees are there to protect the institutional status quo at all cost. The good news is that the really good administrators and far-sighted physicians know that to follow the easy route of maintaining the status quo is a losing proposition in the long term.

If we are to successfully transform America's resource-depleting redundancies in hospitals, it is imperative that trustees adhere to their fundamental responsibilities for governing and deciding about fundamental purpose. My first reading of Chapter Eleven left me railing against Johnson's failure to sound a clarion call for more responsible governance. My second reading left me feeling that he demonstrated that needed changes could not occur because boards do not, perhaps cannot, challenge the status quo. My third reading led me to decide that his assessment of the industry is probably correct, but since I think the status quo is fundamentally flawed the least I could do was to respond that I think we will fail as a profession if we cannot recognize, articulate, and promote a more sound view of the role of governance in the fundamental purpose of the hospital enterprise.

Establishing Purpose and Mission

No one can argue that hospitals are not facing major and fundamental changes in roles, mission, and purpose. Johnson asked, "What is the purpose of hospital governance?" In my estimation, in a very real sense the major purpose is and always has been to *establish* purpose. This is even more the case in troubled times than in times when hospitals are moving along with their chosen activities without much challenge. Today, a board adds little of value if it does not reflect deeply and carefully about purpose, mission, values, and similar issues.

The role of governance is to deliberate and decide on the purpose, mission, and values to be served by an institution. This governance role is always primary, but it becomes more active and critical during times of great environmental change. It is backed up by the corporation's governing laws and is normally articulated in the founding documents of the corporation. Making decisions about such issues may be successfully constrained by the interests of others (physicians, administrators, and individual board members) whose livelihoods are dependent upon the existing articulation of the hospital's purpose, but the final responsibility for answering the ultimate questions of the hospital's purpose and existence rests with trustees. Being constrained, even checkmated, does not change the ultimate responsibility: only a board can vote to close a hospital, sell it, or merge it; only a board can fundamentally change the mission of a hospital. Market forces may change what hospitals do when a board and management default on their responsibilities to anticipate and make changes in order to maintain long-range viability of an institution, but the buck stops with the board when it comes to keeping or changing the institution's fundamental purpose.

Johnson asserts that the primary responsibility of the hospital's board is to perpetuate the institution's existence. Therefore, "it must deal primarily with strategic issues rather than with operational matters." Grand strategy deals fundamentally with purpose, and purpose is at issue today more than at any time in recent memory. Johnson makes this point, but only in passing; it is hardly the central focus of the chapter, which deals much more with peripheral issues related to governance.

Johnson recognizes the important role of governance when he asserts that a hospital must adhere to goals defined within the context of what it wants to do in a community, "unless the governing board elects to adopt a different value system, as did the Mayo Foundation, the Cleveland Clinic, the Columbia Health System, or Kaiser-Permanente." This comment is buried in a chapter that struggles to find a meaningful role of value-added work for governance in today's turbulent market. By not dealing fully with this important role, Johnson's comments about governance having very little to do with decisions in running PHOs and managed care obscure the more vital point of what governance is really all about, and obscure its centrality in deciding how, fundamentally, to deal with physicians and managed care. Governance is about purpose, and nothing is more important today than sorting out just how the assets of hospitals should be deployed within a system of care that makes hospitals cost centers rather than revenue centers.

Do Boards Add Value?

Johnson sorts through a number of issues to ascertain whether or not trustees add value. Managed care, pricing, competition, credentialing, and other issues, he rightly contends, get resolved mainly by others in the hospital. It is true that many boards of trustees actually are adrift in such matters and seem not to know just what their role is or should be. As I suspect, many do not understand that their main role is to decide just how they should act in order to position the hospital in the changing health care environment.

Johnson's discussion of individual assessments of value added is clear, and definitely add value to that process. In fact, too little has been written about the process of looking hard at evaluating individual trustees.

At the macro, strategic level, boards have great responsibilities and much to offer. Some boards do in fact make major contributions to managed care, mergers, networking, and the like. But they do not do it by meddling in operations; they do it through their contribution to deciding how best to position the hospital to be a player in a larger system. For example, a hospital in Central Florida decided that the future of the industry was going to be shaped more and more by managed care. Rather than bemoaning that fact, the hospital authorized the establishment of what is now a very successful, statewide managed care company. They own the managed care company, which in many respects acts more like a parent to the hospital than vice versa. This is action on purpose. The original concept of hospital as purpose was too restrictive; managed care is much broader. In both concepts, the health needs of the community are being met.

In another instance, a hospital board decided that the future was going to hold more and more deleterious competition among too many community hospitals. The board sold the hospital and established a foundation that today spends tens of millions of dollars each year on the kinds of charitable activities that motivated its founders. The hospital is in the thick of competition, with its new owner spending hundreds of millions of dollars to keep it going. The trustees focused on a fundamental purpose, sought options to configuration and use of resources, acted accordingly, and ensured that their larger purpose would guide them into the future.

Governance in Managed Care

This decade is witnessing the rapid growth of managed care, with more and more entities putting real pressure on hospitals and physicians to compete based on price. In the day-to-day working out of relationships, board members have less of a role than they might desire in decisions on programs, credentialing, and other issues. To a certain extent, it seems that Johnson sees this decreased role as detracting from the value that trustees play in the activities of the institution.

Because I see the governance responsibility as being primarily one of managing purpose and secondarily one of providing oversight and evaluation of management, it would seem that the opportunity to add value to a hospital is greatly enhanced during times of fundamental change. True, boards do not and probably should not have operational or quasi-operational decision-making responsibility. But they have a large role in planning the strategic role of the organization.

What are the implications that managed care presents to the purpose of the hospital? Is a single- or multiple-hospital entity the better way to deploy resources? Should the hospital add PHOs, employ physicians, buy a managed care company, join a network, or sell the hospital to another network? How can its underlying charter or purpose best be furthered? This is serious work. This is relevant work. And it is very much needed in today's health care environment.

Within this larger frame of reference, it would be entirely possible, perhaps highly desirable, for hospital trustees to deliberately transform the hospital asset base into a vertically integrated entity with large managed care and physician components. This can happen and will happen where boards take seriously their responsibilities for managing purpose.

The Role of Governance in Mergers and Consolidation

Johnson noted that board members "find it difficult to make a decision to merge when the only outcome is a loss of value." He further noted that the "two driving forces of a hospital governing board are to add value to the functioning of the organization and to perpetuate the hospital's existence." If one views the role of governance as primarily perpetuating the hospital's current use of assets and resources, then the mergers and consolidations needed to build effective regional, vertically integrated organizations are going to come very slowly. If, however, one views governance as fundamentally in the business of continually managing the purpose of the organization, one must also view the assets of the organization not as fundamental embodiments of purpose but merely as the configuration needed to implement a former decision about purpose. If assets are separate from purpose, then a hospital company could easily liquidate its assets and become a foundation or managed care company. Some towns have sold hospitals and used the proceeds to build sewers and water treatment plants. The purpose of health is served by both uses of assets. Other owners now sell the hospital service, while the towns sell water and sewer services. Today's business mode of hospital operation is not as close to the public purpose of towns as these other services. In the case of not-for-profit hospitals, selling the hospital is a logical extension of the desire to employ resources to meet the fundamental purpose of the owners or trustees. Where no original owners or founders exist with any reserved rights over purpose, the successors are fully empowered to decide on the purpose and on the population they deem to be the appropriate beneficiaries of asset deployment and use.

Having taken the opportunity to reflect on some ideas about governance and to use Richard Johnson's chapter on the purpose of hospital governance as a vehicle to that end, I commend his chapter to all readers. Johnson always adds to my thinking on subjects, even when I do not agree with him.

Johnson's Response

As I had anticipated, Monty Brown has provided a thoughtful and articulate commentary on the ideas expressed in Chapter Eleven. He has been a respected colleague and friend for many years. Both of us have enjoyed our differing thoughts on many topics. We look forward to including a wide circle of our professional friends in a discussion on this subject.

From a personal perspective, I am supportive of the vision of the role of the hospital Brown described in his commentary. With all my heart, I would like to see it happen. However, we part ways over the question of what hospitals *will* do versus what hospitals *should* do." My thoughts are based on what I believe most hospitals *will* do.

As I understand Brown's position, he assumes that the majority of hospitals will be able to transform themselves into organizations with a more comprehensive role that encompasses such nontraditional hospital activities as prepayment, managed care, and physician practices. My belief is to the contrary. The driving force for both physicians and hospitals in responding to a payer-dominated marketplace will be to form integrated delivery systems. To successfully compete for managed care contracts, the integrated delivery systems will be dependent upon clinical and managerial knowledge, supported by a well-developed management information system. The front line of decision making for providers will shift from the hospital boardroom to a new organization dominated by clinical and management viewpoints blended together for negotiating purposes. The role of the hospital will become secondary.

In my judgment, the governing boards of most nonprofit hospitals are not apt to undergo the transformation Brown believes will take place. Board members are likely to continue to view themselves as representatives of the community and to remain unpaid trustees. These deeply rooted concepts are so ingrained that they will remain in place even though the health care environment will continue to change markedly. As a result, hospital governing boards will gradually lose more and more influence on the events occurring in health care. Over time, the power they have possessed will erode and shift to the organized delivery system dominated by physicians and hospital executives in a new corporate setting. The inability of hospital governing boards to go beyond their traditional role will make them peripheral to the required decision making. Governing boards will belatedly recognize that the name of the new game is professional competence, not voluntary trusteeship.

Brown's Response

Richard Johnson and I differ far less than either of us might have thought as we began this exercise. My reading of Johnson's response to my comments is as follows:

1.   My expectations are that more integrated systems will develop than Johnson believes. These systems will include the nontraditional activities of prepayment, managed care, and physician practices. These activities are not distinct from the integrated system; they define the integrated system.

2.   Johnson sees these systems as developing outside the governance structure of not-for-profit hospitals. True, it is happening that way, with the hospital assets being shifted to organizations that have less and less control by communities. The assets of the not-

for-profit hospitals and of the traditional Blue Cross plans and not-for-profit HMOs are being shifted to these new for-profit operations in which physicians and managers are more and more likely to be rewarded with stock (equity) positions, which ultimately gives them an incentive to actually sell off the operations to even larger stock companies down the road.

3. Both Johnson and I see the same things happening. Integration is needed to achieve the incentives for efficiency. If it is done as it is being done today, the ultimate end point will be a conversion of assets on a gargantuan scale from community-controlled to equity-market-controlled health care organizations.

4. Our differences are in how we focus our energies and commentary. My efforts are directed at helping communities to restructure in ways that can retain community control and influence over health affairs. Some organizations are doing this and do retain substantial control at the trustee level. Those hospitals that fail to do this will become owned entities controlled by those who do make the transition. The winners will be regional systems with regional boards.

5. If professionals do indeed believe that community control is a virtue worth saving, then it seems that one obligation of health care executives is to find ways to help communities modify their organizations so that they will succeed in the future—for example, helping them to transition to regional organizations where the community is not the local town of origin of the first hospital but the region in which the integrated organization provides comprehensive services to a population of a million or so people.

6. As others join in this debate, perhaps we can sort out the trends and find the ways in which we need to adapt to retain desirable values, while moving to meet the challenge of integrated health organizations.

Chapter Thirteen

Hospital Governance in a Competitive Environment

Richard L. Johnson

Traditionally, nonprofit hospitals regard themselves as institutions that provide community health care services through a form of organization whose year-end profits are ultimately used for reinvestment in capital programs for buildings and equipment and for supporting charity care. As part of this mandate, governing board members typically receive no payment for their services, and because they neither take pay nor benefit from year-end profits, they see themselves as serving the community good through their voluntary efforts. The reward for serving as a volunteer board member of a nonprofit hospital comes from knowing that one is participating in directing a vital community service. In a bygone era, board participation required not only one's time, but might well include contributing substantial sums of money to undertake building-expansion programs or to offset a year-end operating deficit.

In days past, hospitals were not major employers in their communities, nor did they have budgets that were among the largest in town. Following World War II, hospitals were just beginning to be recognized as an essential community service. This recognition led to the passage of the Hill-Burton Act by Congress, which provided substantial funds for building and expanding community hospitals, with particular concern for rural and semirural areas of the country. Competition among hospitals was nonexistent. Most hospitals had average occupancies of more than ninety percent, and during the winter months they would add hall beds to hold overflow patients until regular accommodations became available through the discharge of other patients. Hospital governance focused on finding money to provide the wherewithal to keep up with the need for facilities and equipment. Community fund drives were commonplace, and the financial acumen required to deal with expansion programs was provided by board members.

Expansion plans for additional beds were determined by an administrator, who scanned the number of patients on the waiting list for admission and estimated how many beds should be added, usually in increments the size of nursing units, which might be from twenty-four to thirty beds per unit. If the administrator's estimate was overstated, it was not of any serious consequence; the opening of the new unit would simply be delayed for up to a year to allow the demand for additional beds to catch up with the supply. Making the right decision was a relatively easy task. Errors in judgment by the administrator or in the decisions of the governing board were quickly bypassed and had no lasting impact. Time healed every mistake.

The Shifting Medical Scene

By 1994, the hospital world had changed markedly. Table 13.1 compares a typical two-hundred-bed hospital in 1950 with a typical two-hundred-bed hospital in 1994, revealing the transformation that has taken place. If revenues in 1950 were five percent less than operating expenses at year-end, the governing board was expected to cover the deficit—in this case, $65,700. By 1994, if the hospital had an operating loss of five percent, the gap between revenue and expense would be $2.628 million, a fortyfold increase over 1950, and an amount unlikely to be covered by passing a hat around the board table.

Since 1950, technology has increasingly become the engine of progress. To keep up with the accompanying demands placed on the hospital organization, the management staff has grown accordingly. The senior management of 1950 consisted of an administrator and perhaps an assistant administrator. By 1994, senior management consisted of a sophisticated, in-depth, experienced group of ten to fifteen people. Their skills in their respective

**Table 13.1. Comparison of Operating Results of a
Two-Hundred-Bed Hospital in 1950 and 1994.**

Year	1950	1994
Number of beds	200	200
Number of full-time employees	360	900
Average number of patients	180	120
Average occupancy rate	90 percent	60 percent
Annual adjusted patient days	65,700	44,019
Average cost per day	$20	$800
Annual cost of operations		
Inpatient	$1.314M	$35.215M
Outpatient	—	$17.345M
Total operating cost	$1.314M	$52.560M

spheres of management collectively far exceeded those of the governing board with respect to knowledge of the health field, its trends, and its financing.

While these changes were taking place in management, equally important changes were occurring medically. Clinical specialization proliferated to the point where in 1994 70 percent of practicing physicians were specialists. To cope with their clinical needs, hospitals have increasingly allocated space, equipment, and technically trained personnel to provide the necessary support. For the past fifteen years, specialists have been developing new techniques for the diagnosis and treatment of many diseases and injuries that could safely be performed on an ambulatory basis. This trend has added greatly to the complexity of the hospital organization because patients are now seen on both an inpatient and outpatient basis. Hospitals that originally were built to provide services to patients on a horizontal plane have had to be remodeled or replaced in order to provide services to patients on a vertical plane as well.

As the breadth of services increased, the money required to support these activities also grew at a rapid clip. Health care spending grew from 5 percent of the gross domestic product (GDP) in 1950 to 14 percent in 1994, and it is projected to increase to 17 percent by 2000, with total health care expenditures projected to be $1.7 trillion. Thus, fueled by clinical specialization and the accompanying technological explosion, health care expenditures have increased faster than the rate of inflation, and government and business have decried the annual increases in premium costs they have had to pay for health care coverage for employees.

The Technological Enterprise

Until recently, health care was provider dominated, but it is in the throes of becoming purchaser dominated. Providers are increasingly being forced to compete for contracts to provide services, both ambulatory and inpatient. Competition is intensifying as large blocs of patient care are put up for bidding by the purchasers of health care services.

In this increasingly competitive environment, voluntary hospital governing boards that serve the community's interests are discovering that the decisions that need to be made are concerned with the needs of a capitalistic free market, not with the needs of the overall community. Of overriding interest is the necessity of protecting the investment for which board members are responsible. Today, a typical hospital is a technological enterprise with a budget of more than $50 million, a capital investment in buildings and equipment of more than $55 million, and often an outstanding debt of $15 to $20 million. Board members recognize that the protection of that asset is their primary responsibility. Of necessity, if a community health need is unfulfilled, or inadequately fulfilled, and can reach only a break-even point in terms of revenue, it will probably be ignored. Where competition exists there is the added incentive of commencing new programs and services before other local hospitals see the same opportunities and move in first. As a result, there is unnecessary duplication of facilities and programs because hospitals fear loss of market share or are attempting to offset a financial mix of patients that is adverse to the hospital's financial interests.

Hospital board members agree to duplicate facilities and programs because of administrative recommendations or in response to physician requests. Since physicians are not economically tied to the hospital, their desires for new programs or equipment are based on enhancing their clinical diagnostic or treatment skills, or for providing an additional opportunity for professional fee enhancement, or both. There is usually a secondary concern about the hospital's ability to, in the process, either break even or profit from adding the activity. Caught in the middle are governing boards, who reluctantly approve unnecessary duplication because of physician clinical interests or administrative concerns about losing market share. In deciding whether to make a decision that is for the good of the community or good for the hospital, board members are keenly aware that they have to come down on the side of protecting the interests of the hospital and the medical staff.

Why do hospital governing boards approve the unnecessary duplication of facilities if they see themselves as representatives of community interests? Clearly, they have the authority to reject recommendations. On balance, it has to be concluded that governing board members believe that the perpetuation of their hospital as a viable technological organization outweighs any concerns they might have about community good.

The Role of the Hospital

A similar set of circumstances is now arising with regard to wellness programs. Speakers addressing hospital audiences are proclaiming that the community hospital has to introduce organized programs to promote wellness among the public, that the way for hospitals to contain health care costs is to lead the way by undertaking wellness activities. On the surface, such a plea seems reasonable, since wellness is a desirable social goal. No one can oppose the idea of a healthier citizenry. However, it is important to look more deeply at this subject and inquire whether this is really a role for the community hospital, or whether the responsibility more properly belongs to some other organization.

The hospital's role, and the role of physicians on a medical staff is to provide both diagnostic and treatment services to the sick and injured. A distinction needs to be made, however, about physicians. When primary care physicians refer patients to specialists, it is because they believe the patient has a condition requiring treatment; in other words, something needs to be fixed and they (as primary care physicians) believe that the specialist is in the best position to provide this type of service, with the hospital backing up the specialist's skills as required. Conversely, the primary care physician is rightfully concerned about wellness, because he or she is in the unique position of advising patients about the best ways to stay healthy, and being paid for it through office visit fees or capitation. It is in both the patient's and the primary care physician's best interests to keep the patient in good health.

By contrast, the hospital's role is not to promote wellness but to provide a place for the treatment of disease. Hospital revenues are, and should be, spent for this purpose. This is an important activity that is essential to a community. So is wellness, but the organizational and financial support for wellness properly lies in the domain of prepayment plans, particularly within the framework of managed care. Prepayment plans that use capitation stand to gain financially by keeping their subscribers healthy and out of the hands of the specialist and the hospital. To the degree that capitation succeeds with wellness programs, managed care plans stand to enhance their bottom lines. The costs for wellness activities should be borne by those organizations that stand to profit from keeping patients away from specialists.

An easy way to appreciate these relationships is to apply an analogy. If one thinks of a hospital as a garage and specialists as mechanics, it is not in the best interests of the garage or the mechanics to publicly promote preventive maintenance programs that reduce the flow of customers. However, it is in the best interests of the automobile manufacturer to develop cars that require fewer and fewer trips to a service department or garage because the reputations of such cars will increase sales. Because governing board members see their role as serving the community good, they may be prone to approve funding for wellness and fail to appreciate that these incurred expenses become an additional burden when bidding on a managed care contract. In a competitive environment, staying lean and mean requires careful scrutiny of all expenses and the elimination of those that do not directly contribute to the ongoing activities of the organization. This means that hospitals should not take on a responsibility that will work against them when bidding for a managed care contract.

Wellness properly belongs on the managed care plan's expense statement.

Capitating Payments to Hospitals

It is now fashionable to claim that in a capitated payment system a hospital is an expense center and not a revenue center, but this is only partially correct. If the hospital is owned by the prepayment organization, then the hospital is a cost center and the fewer patients it admits, the greater will be the net income to the parent corporation. Under capitation, keeping patients away from hospitals and specialists is important because the number of patients will impact the managed care plan's ability to offer a premium rate to subscribers that is competitive in the marketplace.

However, when a community hospital is not owned by the prepayment organization but contracts with it for the provision of services, the relationship between the prepayment organization and the hospital is quite different. Competition enters the picture when the hospital bids against competing hospitals for a contract to provide services for a managed care organization. In this setting, the bid submitted by the hospital to the managed care organization is evaluated on a price basis—the lower the price, the more likely the hospital is to win the contract. In a bidding situation, it does not matter whether the unit of payment is capitation, payment per admission, per diem payment, or a discount of charges; what matters is that the bid be lowest, whatever the method of payment. The buyer's interest is the reverse, to obtain the best price. The aim of the hospital is to win the contract at the highest possible price, since the hospital is seeking to maximize its revenue.

Even under capitation, the aim of a contracted hospital is to maximize revenue. It could be argued that capitation benefits hospitals that keep patient services to a minimum, or by supporting wellness programs to keep patients out of the hospital. However, this is only a short-term gain because the managed care plan undoubtedly will recognize that it is paying more than necessary, and at the end of the contract period it will renegotiate capitation downward to a level more favorable to its own interests.

Hospital governing boards, which are imbued with the concept of community good, need to appreciate that the growth of managed care only increases competition among the providers and pushes community interests into the background. The goal of managed care is to tightly control payments to hospitals and physicians, since such payments represent an expense to the managed care organization. Community good and wellness programs are worthwhile for prepayment organizations only to the extent that they reduce payments to providers and thereby provide a greater margin of profit. Managed care focuses on the tangible dollar benefits arising out of competition, not on community good. This focus in turn forces the providers to play by the same rules, like it or not. When the majority of health care is paid for by managed care plans, community good disappears.

The Role of the Governing Board

Where does the hospital governing board fit into this developing competitive climate? If by not accepting money for serving as a board member the tie to community service remains strong and the hospital is linked to its previous role as a charitable institution, is value added to the functioning of the hospital? Or does this approach lead to a loss of value in the functioning of the hospital? Or is a redefinition of the traditional role of governance needed in order to add value? If community good has been replaced with intense competition and the charitable institution has been replaced with a technological enterprise, what is needed to ensure governing board effectiveness?

Board effectiveness is largely determined by individual board members' actions as they discuss and vote on issues. The matters they act upon should reflect their perceptions of their role. This does not seem to be the case, however. In reviewing the types of decisions hospital governing boards make in terms of whether they add value or subtract value (see Table 13.2), it is evident that their actions reflect a view of themselves as board members of a technological enterprise. Yet, if asked to describe their role, they are most likely to say that they represent the community and are primarily concerned with approving programs and making decisions that are in the best interests of community health. They do not say that they make decisions on the basis of what adds or subtracts value in the functioning of the institution. Their feelings reflect

Table 13.2. Hospital Governing Board Perceptions of Value.

Adding Value	Losing Value
Acquiring another hospital	Being mergered into another hospital
Commencing a new clinical program	Dropping an existing clinical program
Renovating and remodeling space	Closing nursing units
Reducing bad debts	Increasing bad debts
Reducing days in accounts receivable	Increasing days in accounts receivable
Making more annual profit than budgeted	Making less annual profit than budgeted
Increasing patient days/ admissions	Decreasing patient days/ admissions
Successful bidding for managed care contract	Unsuccessful bidding for managed care contract
Adding physicians to medical staff	Losing physicians from medical staff
Adding health related services (such as DME-Home Health)	Closing health related services
Adding personnel	Laying off personnel
Winning a lawsuit	Losing a lawsuit
Operating at a profit	Operating at a loss
Favorable media reporting	Unfavorable media reporting
Taking on major long-term debt	Inability to meet loan payment schedule
Buying land for hospital expansion	Selling hospital land at a loss
Purchasing sophisticated capital equipment	Inability to provide latest technology
Successful community fund drive	Poor results from community fund drive
Budget projection held at GDP	Budget projection exceeds GDP
Establishing off-site services	Closing off-site services
Retaining complete autonomy	Partially giving up autonomy
Successful physician-hospital integration	Lack of support for physician-hospital integration

their social concerns and are reinforced by their not taking a salary for performing their duties. Yet, board decisions support a corporation that is both labor and capital intensive, and a major economic force in its local community.

As managed care grows and becomes the dominant form of payment to hospitals, the environment of health care will inevitably become more intensely competitive. Governing board decisions in such a climate will of necessity become more and more pragmatic, forcing social concerns and the hospital's role of serving the community good to become less and less relevant. The public clearly understands that the role of the hospital and of specialist physicians is to cure illness and alleviate pain. The court system also recognizes this role, as does the public. Both the courts and the public hold providers to standards for diagnosing and treating illness, not standards of social responsibility. In a highly competitive marketplace in which the low-bidding provider is the success story, social concerns are either lost or diminished.

Affiliating to Bid on Managed Care

As hospitals are forced to bid for managed care contracts, will they be able to bring to the negotiating table enough economic leverage to enable them to deal as equals with the managed care organizations they face? Concern about this is already evident, as hospitals in the same general area affiliate or network with one another in order to offer the managed care plan an in-place arrangement, which may also include physician organizations. By representing broad geographic areas, these affiliations are attempting to make themselves attractive to managed care plans, which need to be able to offer care to employers whose employees live in a widely dispersed area. (These affiliations are not sufficiently concentrated, however, to run the risk of antitrust problems.)

Participation in an affiliated organization is attractive to hospital governing boards. On the surface, affiliations appear to offer a number of advantages without corresponding disadvantages. For example, to become an affiliate, a hospital does not have to relinquish any of its decision-making authority. If the governing board, for whatever reasons, decides that it is no longer desirable for the hospital to participate, they can elect to withdraw, without any penalty for doing so, a fact that is often viewed positively by governing boards and chief executives.

However, the ability to withdraw at any time is a serious flaw, which is often overlooked in making a decision to affiliate, and not usually discovered until much later. The inability to hold a group together leads affiliations to crumble under the stress of competition. If one of the member hospitals elects to bid for a contract outside of the affiliation because it determines that it might thus be able to capture a much larger share of the managed care market, the remaining affiliates are inevitably forced to do the same thing in order to protect their own interests. In addition, it should be anticipated that managed care plans will attempt to deal with individual members of an affiliation, to offer them a larger bloc of patients than they would receive as part of the affiliation—a temptation that will be hard for hospitals to resist. The managed care plan may well consider such attempts to split apart an affiliated group of hospitals to be in the interest of the community, whether it actually is or not, because the community is concerned with achieving the lowest possible price from providers. A hospital governing board may be imbued with the spirit of community good, but when faced with a take-it-or-leave-it situation, the financial imperatives of the hospital will dictate the results.

Three Phases of Hospital Governance

Over the past three-quarters of a century, hospital governing boards have undergone a subtle shift of viewpoint, one that has occurred so gradually that it has barely been noticed by governing boards. In the first half of the twentieth century, governing boards acted as charitable, nonprofit organizations, rarely having much of a bottom line, and largely content with knowing that at the end of the fiscal year the hospital had broken even in its finances. This era was followed by the development of hospitals into technological enterprises. Because of the movement in medicine away from general practice into specialty fields, supported by an ever-increasing sophistication of diagnostic and treatment equipment, the hospital found itself having to make larger and larger investments in its facilities, equipment, and specialized personnel. Huge increases in the cost of operations occurred year after year, using up not only any reserve or surplus funds, but requiring substantial long-term debt just to keep up with the latest developments.

In the latter stage of this era, clinical know-how and technology led to the ability to provide more and more kinds of care on an ambulatory basis, once again requiring huge sums of money to retrofit physical facilities to accommodate this development. Over the years, the charitable nature of the hospital lost out to technology. The desire to meet community need was redefined as the ability to provide the best, the latest, and the most comprehensive range of services possible. Competition steadily increased as each hospital tried to provide more services than the other hospitals in the community. The result was an "arms" race (which continues to this day) in which cost was a secondary concern. Hospital governing boards interpreted their responsibility as providing their communities with the best medical care possible, and chose to define community interest in these terms as well. The result was an outstanding success. The charitable institution of the early years that primarily offered nursing care and limited surgery turned into a technological enterprise that today is recognized worldwide as offering the best diagnostic and treatment technology available— clearly, the world leader. The hospital as we now know it is the result of separate forces that ultimately meet at the front door of the hospital.

Advanced engineering and computers led the way for advances in equipment. Specialty training led to the widespread capability of physicians, and the development of graduate programs for hospital executives resulted in experienced, well-trained managers. To some extent, these developments were augmented by the hospitals' nonprofit status and by their not having to pay corporate or property taxes, which meant more money could be used for capital investment.

The third era has only recently commenced and is in its early stages of development. Today, the modern hospital is recognized publicly as an essential community service. It is so important that it is regarded as a necessity that must be readily available to everyone, irrespective of the ability to pay. The issue now before the public has nothing to do with whether hospitals and physicians are able to provide high-level, sophisticated treatment. The issue is now one of being able to pay for health care resources.

It now appears that the two eras of provider dominance are being replaced with an era of payer dominance. The theme of the future is competition through managed care. Managed care plans, corporate self-funded plans, and governmental plans are all seeking ways to limit annual increases in health care expenditures. Because health care consistently has outpaced the GDP year after year, the payers have concluded that the most effective way to restrict these increases is to make one monthly payment per individual or family, for which each patient will receive as much care as needed and which will put the providers collectively "at risk." The payers assume that this method will force both hospitals and physicians to become more efficient because the revenues they receive will be fixed and will not vary by the amount of services provided.

In this developing climate, hospital governing boards will once again be forced to find a new role. What began as an overriding focus on charitable undertakings and then became a focus on technological development must now shift to a focus on successfully competing for business in an increasingly competitive marketplace. The role of the governing board will largely be that of a bystander. Successfully competing for a managed care contract will depend on clinical and managerial knowledge, supported by a well-developed management information system. The front line of decision-making will shift from the boardroom to the administrative suite, where clinical and management viewpoints will be blended together for negotiating purposes.

Responding to the payer's interest in having a bundled package of physician and hospital services for one price will lead to the demise of hospital affiliations based on collectively negotiating for hospital services only. The integration of physician and hospital services into one package will be, and already is, favored by payers. Out of this need for hospitals and physicians to respond with one voice, a new organizational form will develop. This organizational structure will in many cases be outside of the hospital and will become the most powerful health care entity because of its role in securing managed care contracts. Given the depth and type of knowledge required to negotiate with managed care plans, these new organizations will most likely have governing boards dominated by experienced health care professionals from the clinical and administrative ranks. In all probability, these new organizational entities will become models for other health care providers who have not yet reached that stage of development.

Alternative Organizational Structures

The development of separate physician-hospital organizations into integrated provider delivery systems is likely to be only one form of response to managed care. Because of the difficulties inherent in bringing independent physicians and a hospital together into one organization, other developments will also take place. Until managed care is a substantial threat in a local community, many physicians are unlikely to opt to participate. The hospital, however, may be of a different mind-set. Wanting to protect its assets, it may seek to merge or consolidate with other area hospitals, believing that a system of hospitals has advantages over freestanding institutions. Governing boards often see this as a first step. However voluntary, nonprofit hospital boards usually have a strong distaste for any arrangement that requires a loss of total autonomy, unless the financial viability of the institution is threatened.

Other hospitals are looking in the direction of purchasing the practices of physicians, preferably primary care physicians. This approach is viewed as a way of assuring a flow of patients without impacting the decision-making autonomy of the governing board. Even within nonprofit systems of hospitals that have been in existence for a decade or longer, the question of autonomy is a nagging problem. Money earned at the local level is often regarded as available only for capital expenditures at the hospital where it was earned and as not to be transferred in toto to the corporate office for reallocation to another hospital in the same system. It is clear that nonprofit hospital governing boards favor arrangements or purchases that do not impinge on the institution's authority and that leave the hospital in control of its own destiny. Viewing their role as community representatives, as board members do, and not being paid for their services work against aggregating health care resources into one organizational structure and inhibit the development of large economic units.

Facing the Future

It can be anticipated that in the years ahead the most important decisions facing the hospital will be the negotiations it conducts for contracts with managed care plans. These negotiations will become more and more technical. The third-party payers increasingly will concern themselves with both clinical outcomes and the costs of the services rendered to patients. Negotiations will involve both elements. In the emerging payer-driven environment, hospitals and physicians will be required to jointly bid on books of business by submitting a one-price bid. As a result of the need to bid against competitor groups, financial decisions will be controlled by the organization of physicians and hospitals, not by the hospital alone, as has been true in the past. Not only will financial decisions shift out of the hospital, but to a large extent so will the credentialing of physicians, since they will be evaluated on both the clinical and economic factors of their practice.

With a few years of experience, these new entities will have smoothed out their operations and will be apt to seek new opportunities. Recognizing the potential for greater financial returns, they most likely will turn their attention toward capitation, and perhaps become "at risk." This will have to be done by for-profit rather than nonprofit organizations. Carried to the ultimate extreme, an organization that uses capitation and becomes successful will in turn probably want to have as a "captive" hospital the one with which it is affiliated. It appears that the model for the future will be a corporate health care entity that incorporates prepayment, a hospital, and physicians. Whether the control of this corporate entity stems from the hospital or the physicians or the managed care plan will depend on which component is the most aggressive. Which component wins out will vary from one community to another. While the desire of each component may be to hold the winning hand, the controlling elements are the competitive forces at work in the marketplace.

If present trends and public attitudes prevail, the future of health care in the United States will be determined primarily by the premium paid per member per month. Considerations of quality, range of health care services available, and physician capability will be of secondary importance to those making the buying decisions. This will be a bitter pill to swallow for both hospitals and physicians, who have always been concerned primarily with the quality of care. Doing the best that can be done for each individual patient has been the hallmark of the American medical care system, but under managed care the right of the individual to freely select a physician and hospital gives way to price considerations. Even if the members of a given plan encounter bad experiences with the health care services available to them, the decision to seek another managed care plan will also depend on the price tag. Price is always the most important consideration until one has more than enough money, and then it's service that counts.

Conclusions

The scenario I have described does not support the vision of the hospital remaining the dominating force in health care. It would be nice to have the hospital continue as the centerpiece. However, when examining the question of what hospitals *will* do versus what hospitals *should* do, some see a much more expanded role for hospitals, while others expect the hospital role to decrease in importance.

Unfortunately, it can be concluded from experience that the majority of hospitals will be unable to transform their role into a more comprehensive one that encompasses the nontraditional hospital activities of prepayment, managed care, and physician practices. The driving force for both physicians and hospitals in responding to a payer-dominated marketplace will be to form integrated delivery systems in which clinical and managerial knowledge will be paramount in decision making. This will shift the front line of providers' decision making away from the hospital boardroom to a new organization in which clinical and managerial viewpoints will blend together for negotiating purposes. The role of the hospital will become secondary.

Most nonprofit hospital governing boards are not apt to undergo the necessary transformation. Board members are likely to continue to view themselves as representatives of the community and to remain unpaid trustees. These concepts are so deeply ingrained that they will remain in place even though the health care environment will be markedly changed. As a result, hospital governing boards will gradually lose more and more influence on the events occurring in health care. Over time, the power they have possessed will erode and shift to the new corporate entities dominated by physicians and hospital executives. The inability of hospital governing boards to move beyond their traditional role will make them peripheral to the required decision making. Belatedly, governing boards will recognize that the name of the new game is professional competence, not voluntary trusteeship, as illustrated by the changing perceptions of value shown in Table 13.2.

Chapter Fourteen

Competition, Managed Care, and Trusteeship

Can Voluntary Hospital Governance Survive? Will Not-for-Profit Hospitals Survive?

Montague Brown

Chapter Thirteen, "Hospital Governance in a Competitive Environment," makes the case for a major disconnection between what trustees of voluntary hospitals currently do and what they will do when faced with the question of survival of the institutions they represent. While the chapter does not explicitly predict the demise of the voluntary hospital in the United States, it is difficult to accept the developments portended and the continued existence of the voluntary community hospitals in their present form, serving the community interests.

Is this likely to be a correct analysis? Blue Cross plans across the country are considering entering into equity markets to raise capital and putting their best managed care products into such enterprises. These plans, too, have evolved from the not-for-profit community-benefit type of organization. Over time, Blue Cross and Blue Shield are evolving into commercial enterprises driven in

Note: This chapter has been adapted from Brown, M. "Commentary: Competition, Managed Care, and Trusteeship: Can Voluntary Hospital Governance Survive? Will Not-for-Profit Hospitals Survive?" *Health Care Management Review,* 1995, *20*(1), 84–89. Copyright © 1995, Aspen Publishers, Inc. Used with permission.

large part by their attention to profits and stock values. More and more public and voluntary hospital boards have elected the exit strategy of selling the hospital to other organizations, which not infrequently have been for-profit enterprises. In the last few years, these for-profit enterprises have recruited physicians by offering them minority ownership positions in the enterprise. The success of this strategy is best demonstrated by the meteoric rise of Columbia, which took over the hospitals of both Humana and the Hospital Corporation of America, which previously had been the two largest hospital chains in the nation. Some insurers, including Blue Cross, have started looking at owning hospitals as part of their managed care strategies. There can be no doubt that change is afoot.

Is the direction of the industry away from voluntary board control? Will this include the loss of assets and control through a transformation of the industry from not-for-profit to for-profit? It is important to closely examine the arguments in order to test the thesis of a total or near total transformation of the industry to a for-profit, stockholder-owned industry.

The hospital is a technological enterprise. The nature of the most highly sought after services of hospitals are technological. To succeed, hospitals must have volumes of amply compensated cases that appropriately utilize their services. Even under capitation, hospitals must seek the highest level of compensation possible, while buyers desire to pay the lowest price. Too much hospital efficiency only results in managed care organizations lowering their prices on the next round of contracts. Clearly, any hospital that depends on high-tech medicine and that has no strategy for meeting managed care expectations for both high-tech and efficiency will be in trouble.

In order to survive in a highly aggressive managed care environment, hospitals must strike a partnership with physicians through a physician-hospital organization or similar organization in which physicians, managers, and technocrats will jointly negotiate relationships with managed care organizations. Trustees interested in the welfare of the community have no talents to offer in this scenario. Thus, their role and that of the hospital per se will atrophy. If trustees are excluded from this decision-making arena, it will be because they fail to see its significance and/or fail to recompose the board so that it possesses the level of talent needed.

It could turn out that trustees are more capable of this kind of no-nonsense negotiation than similarly capable physicians and hospital administrators.

In addition, the logic of managed care is that lower and lower prices will result in lower and lower cost. Ultimately, this pressure rules out any service that cannot make a positive, immediate contribution to the bottom line. Hospitals can be faulted for investing in wellness programs because they reduce the pathology in the population, which in turn creates less revenue for the hospital. The cost of wellness programs should be borne by managed care organizations because they singularly benefit from reduced pathology. Hospitals profit from pathology and should resist any expense or effort to reduce such pathology. Could such services be offered under managed care? Can we really expect wellness centers from managed care companies, since their profit horizons are measured in weeks and months, not decades? Community organizations have much longer horizons, measured in years. If the public is pushed into the lowest-cost medicine, long-term impacts will not survive. In the rush into managed care, has the community service role already been abandoned?

Hospital executives and physicians can adapt their behavior to these changed circumstances and move ahead to deal effectively with managed care. Hospital trustees will have a much more difficult time abandoning a community mission. If trustees fail, will this be a failure of governance or will it be a failure of hospital executives to prepare trustees for governance in a changed world? If trustees adapt and abandon community and social purpose, will they have succeeded or failed?

Rather than being seen as community organizations, hospitals can be characterized by their activities as organizations that improve the health of the community. This is a very restricted view of organizations. If the determination is ultimately made that it is desirable to create community benefit by changing the character and nature of health care delivery, then organizations can set out to do so. There are ways in which a not-for-profit structure can be retained. Kaiser Permanente comes to mind as a not-for-profit, charitable, community-benefit ownership structure that also delivers health care services in a cost-effective manner. Henry Ford Hospital is continuing its transformation into a health maintenance type organization while maintaining its excellence in high-tech medicine and wellness services. These are two examples of this kind of transformation. Those who have completed this transformation may be exceptions, but that is how the world eventually changes—successful innovations get copied.

Hospitals are now forming networks, but they lack contractual arrangements that lock them in place. Lack of commitment necessarily dooms many networks to failure. Trustees have difficulty accepting this premise, just as health care executives have difficulty subordinating their role to a larger entity. Both trustees and executives must yield if hospitals are to merge and build comprehensive regional systems of service. Those who do so will find their mission changed, but they will still have a mission. Those who do not respond will eventually lose out in the ensuing competition. This is one of the toughest challenges confronting most governing boards. It may also be one of the more important challenges for the long-term viability of community trusteeship in America. No doubt many hospitals, with full support of medical staffs and hospital executives, will fail because they simply cannot or will not subordinate their own feelings to benefit the public interest in their region. This is especially true if merging requires surrendering separateness and autonomy. In fact, the failure of otherwise outstanding hospitals and hospital executives may prove to be a prerequisite for alerting the more timid to the necessity for change.

Many hospitals will fail before those left standing embrace the future and abandon the ways of the past. If community-oriented leadership fails, community benefit and social mission may eventually disappear from medical care altogether. They are clearly at risk today, even in many hospitals where they should be strongest. Managed care and health reformers' insistence on using market forces and profits to drive the system are having a corrosive impact on many hospitals. Suggesting that wellness programs should be eliminated from hospitals because of their negative impact on the bottom line is itself a dramatic and drastic comment not appreciated by those who believe that wellness programs are a hospital responsibility.

There is no technical or structural barrier to hospitals remaining community-minded organizations. The barriers are people and politics, and the profits to be made by those who would benefit from a transformation to a for-profit enterprise. Hospitals have the resources, including financial, legal, and human resources, to be more creative in transforming the traditional community hospital into a more community-minded enterprise using capitation and direct contracting for services to keep the financial incentives in line with community purpose. However, there are several forces that mitigate against this happening.

First, managed care is designed in a manner that emphasizes financial incentives for physicians, hospital administrators, and owners of networks and insurers. The emphasis on financial incentives in the compensation packages of executives has grown in not-for-profit hospitals. Executive compensation increasingly provides for severance buyouts due to mergers and corporate consolidations. Financial incentives may be provided if hospitals are sold, and opportunities are created for stock ownership if they become for-profit enterprises.

Executives of not-for-profit hospitals now see physicians requesting and receiving equity shares in managed care enterprises, and they want to participate as well. Their colleagues working for managed care firms receive such incentives, as do their colleagues in for-profit hospitals. Even members of religious congregations are receiving such incentives. Human nature responds to such incentives, which leads many hospital executives to encourage their hospitals to shift their assets and business opportunities into for-profit enterprises.

Health care reformers often lack an appreciation of just how an emphasis on managed care and the resulting profits affect their communities. Many who have entered health administration careers do so wanting to do good work and serve their fellow citizens. This motivation is subverted when confronted with short-term, quick-profit-oriented wheelers and dealers. What is needed is better thinking about the consequences of the current reform. Representative Pete Stark (D-CA) is pushing for limiting physician ownership in laboratories and expensive diagnostic equipment, but he leaves the barn door open in allowing entire hospitals to participate in joint ventures with local physicians in order to attract and keep business. Such joint ventures are a powerful motivator to induce physicians into pressuring voluntary boards to sell the community hospital.

When hospitals joint venture with physicians is there any doubt that the reason for such ownership is to influence referrals and to discourage competition? Will hospitals that are unwilling or unable to buy physician loyalty be hurt? Hospital executives and trustees often become locked into concepts about the hospital's role in the health care system. If the role is seen as protecting the current activities of the organization, there is little chance that those individuals will see opportunity for hospitals in a managed care environment. Maintaining flexibility and a willingness to change leads to greater opportunities.

Trustees and hospital executives invest a great deal of attention in achieving higher revenues, better profits, expanded patient services and, under managed care, more premium dollars per member per month. More is not always better or more efficient or more profitable. Adding more value and making health care less expensive and more affordable is the public's concern. Swamping social mission with financial imperatives leads to a loss of social mission. Hospital executives and trustees need to be confronted with a picture of the diminishing role of hospital governance and the potential failure of the community hospital. It is not inevitable, but it is the direction in which we are headed unless corrective action takes place.

Physicians, health care executives, and managed care experts are going to attempt to shift profits and resources into the for-profit bailiwick. The community will be the loser. To prevent it from happening, people need to recognize what is happening, make informed judgments about allowing it to happen, and then take action. To a great extent, the policy makers in Washington do not understand what is taking place beyond the Beltway. Policy analysts and politicians simply do not think about the potential unanticipated consequences. It is not mistaken judgment, simply a void. If they did stop to think about it, someone would be at their side to tell them that such change is far-fetched and that if it happened the country might be better off anyway.

Changing the hospital trustee's attitude may be an insurmountable barrier that will nudge the hospital into a for-profit mode for the sake of survival even though community participation may be lost. If the hospital of today is so wedded to its present role that it cannot successfully shift into a managed care environment, it will fail. History is replete with examples of new ways supplanting old ways and old ways dying out. The transformation hospitals ultimately may follow this same path.

A paradigm shift in the direction of managed care and lower cost methods of delivering medical care seems inevitable. The question for the community, the community hospital, and the volunteer trustee is whether they will lead, follow, opt out, or get pushed out.

Is this view of current events overstated, or is it an accurate picture? Hospitals are purposeful organizations. If they have thoughtful and imaginative leadership willing to take risks, the future lies in becoming a regional system that offers health insurance, and in effect making this organization a one-stop shop for health financing and provider services. In the short-term, these organizations will partner with insurers. In the long-term, fully-integrated organizations will emerge and replace these intermediate forms. The future belongs to those with the vision, energy, and perseverance sufficient to survive the traumas that will occur as we move toward this brave new world.

Chapter Fifteen

The Challenges of Governing Integrated Health Care Systems

Richard L. Johnson

Two basic organizational structures are under development as hospitals transform themselves from freestanding institutions into integrated health care delivery systems as a result of what is happening in the marketplace. The rapid development of managed care has led physicians and hospitals to conclude that the best strategy for both of them is to become larger so that they will be able to negotiate on an even playing field with managed care organizations. For-profit hospitals have become for-profit health delivery systems, and nonprofit hospitals have become alliances—or stated in other terms, the for-profits have centralized controls while the alliances are voluntary organizations in which only limited authority is ceded to the integrated health care system (IHCS). The difference between a centrally controlled IHCS and an IHCS that has very restricted authority is substantial.

Both forms of organizational structure view competition in the same light, but they have different approaches to consolidation because their respective orientations are dissimilar. The dissimi-

---

Note: This chapter has been adapted from Johnson, R. L. "Challenges of Governing Integrated Health Care Systems." *Health Care Management Review*, 1995, *20*(4), 80–85. Copyright © 1995, Aspen Publishers, Inc. Used with permission.

larities are important to understand in terms of system development and include the following:

- A for-profit orientation versus a nonprofit orientation
- A vertically and horizontally organized IHCS that consists solely of providers versus the same system with a managed care component
- The role of governance versus the role of senior management
- Providing health care services only versus playing an enlarged role that encompasses communitywide responsibilities for prevention and wellness
- Enforcement of the reserved rights of the parent corporation versus local autonomy
- Acceptance by physicians of a collective role with the IHCS versus individual physician autonomy
- The amount of executive time spent on governing board interrelationships versus the time required to manage a complex organization

Each of these issues stands alone, but they are often interconnected in ways that lead to varying outcomes.

Nonprofit Versus For-Profit

One of the most important considerations is whether the IHCS is for-profit or nonprofit. Leaving aside the fact that the for-profit organization is taxable and the nonprofit is not taxable, the organizational ramifications of the form of ownership are significant. If the IHCS is for-profit, then provision must be made for a return on investment (ROI) to those holding shares of stock. For-profit governing boards believe that the provision of an annual dividend or an increasing value per share of stock has precedence over community good, although both are desirable. Since the ROI is a closely watched indicator, a for-profit IHCS carefully restricts the authority of subsidiary governing boards to make decisions by routinely enforcing the rights that have been reserved for the parent corporation. To ensure that the executives of the subsidiary organizations devote their time and energies to their managerial responsibilities, local boards are most likely to be advisory. Concern about interlocking boards, cross-board relationships, rotation of board members among boards, and spinning up or spinning down as ways of coordinating governance are not matters of significance, since the executives are held accountable for making the organization successful. Controls are centralized because it is the parent corporation that must answer to the investors. To accomplish this end, the number of boards are reduced and limited to advisory roles.

This pattern of simplified board structures and greater responsibility and authority for executives is now being adopted by nonprofit IHCSs as they mature as systems. Geisinger, Samaritan, and Legacy systems are all moving in the direction of relying more on management and less on board structures, even though they are nonprofit.

As a freestanding, nonprofit hospital acquires other health-care-related activities and determines that its future lies in becoming an IHCS, it faces two problems that force consideration of a for-profit status. The physician hospital organization (PHO) will likely be for-profit, since the physician component will seek to replace revenue potentially lost from controls on practice payments by having an opportunity to receive dividends or share in the profits that may result from PHO activities. The desire to be a for-profit organization is enhanced if a for-profit managed care plan is part of the IHCS. Combining a for-profit PHO and a for-profit managed care plan as major participants in an IHCS makes it inevitable that the IHCS will be for-profit. In the event that the IHCS determines that it has to quickly acquire additional health care organizations in order to have a regional presence, depending on the "cash cow" hospital to acquire long-term debt may prove to be inadequate. To accomplish the desired end, equity funding may be the financial vehicle of choice. While the hospital may remain nonprofit, it often will be surrounded organizationally by a parent that is for-profit, a for-profit managed care plan, and a for-profit PHO. Under such circumstances, the philosophy of the IHCS will be dominated by the for-profit frame of mind.

Even if the IHCS remains nonprofit, the parent corporation will have the same problem as the for-profit IHCS when it comes to measuring the performances of the subsidiaries. Can separate and distance criteria be applied, or does the parent governing board use a common denominator to reach conclusions about individual subsidiaries' performance? The common denominator in this type of organization, be it for-profit or nonprofit, is the financial results. Did the subsidiary make or lose money?

Profitability is the foremost criterion because governing boards are continually concerned about the perpetuation of the corporation. As a result, the degree to which the IHCS engages in programs of community good means that this interest is always secondary to that of turning a profit.

When the IHCS is an alliance, no such common denominator is available. As a result, alliances are based on trust, commitment to shared goals, and interdependence. Alliances are therefore weak structures and cannot withstand the types of pressure that may be applied to them by aggressive managed care plans seeking to split apart alliances by offering to increase the volume of patients to selected providers in the same alliance.

Provider IHCSs Versus IHCSs with Managed Care

As an IHCS develops from a freestanding hospital into a vertically and horizontally organized provider system, a decision has to be made about whether to develop its own managed care plan, become part owner of an existing one, or remain as only a provider of health care services. This is a tough question to answer because it requires the executives of the IHCS to determine answers to the following questions:

- If the IHCS starts its own managed care plan, will the other managed care plans in the area continue to contract for provider services offered by the IHCS?
- Are there any managed care plans in the area that will permit investment?
- If an IHCS remains only as a provider, will the managed care plans eventually purchase other providers in the local area and freeze others out?
- Can a provider-only IHCS remain sufficiently competitive to be able to underbid competitors?

If the opportunity exists for the IHCS to own a successful managed care plan, the hospital component becomes a cost center of the larger parent organization. This provides a built-in financial protection against decline in and loss of utilization of the hospital, because such decline may well be offset by increasing profits in the managed care component. However, when the IHCS only encompasses providers, any losses sustained by the hospital due to declining utilization cannot be offset because it is a separate and independent revenue center. Hospitals are cost centers only when they are part of a larger organization, and they are revenue centers when they are unaligned with managed care plans.

The Role of Governance
Versus the Role of Senior Management

Coordination of the activities of a variety of subsidiaries is difficult to accomplish by interrelating governing board structures. Even though the transition of a freestanding hospital into an IHCS is a developmental process, through the acquisition of other providers a point is reached when increasing the number of people on a governing board or adding additional boards becomes a real burden to management. Rather than devoting their time and attention to operational matters that have become increasingly complex, management personnel are forced to divert their efforts to the care and feeding of the board structures and members. Decisions are slowed as a result of having to conform to board meeting schedules, and as a result, marketplace opportunities may be missed. Executives recognize that dealing with multiple boards is an unproductive use of their time and talents, and they will seek ways of shifting decision making into their own hands. As an IHCS matures, these problems will be faced and steps will be taken to simplify board structures.

Conversely, if the IHCS is an alliance of health care providers composed of autonomous units who have banded together on a voluntary basis, the possibility of simplifying board structures may not be available. Joint planning may take place, but the implementation of projects remains in the hands of individual alliance members. The process of decision making is slow and the timing of implementation is uncertain, as are the results. Voluntary alliances do not consolidate balance sheets, so the financing of capital projects depends on each member's ability to handle the obligations it agrees to on behalf of the alliance. This makes alliances weak structures that are likely to have increasing difficulties as competition intensifies in their marketplace.

Provider Only Versus Community Responsibility

The extent to which an IHCS should assume a broad community role is an open question. Many hospitals are supportive of the IHCS having a broad community service mission in which the IHCS addresses the social concerns of poverty, unemployment, housing, and nutrition by working cooperatively with other community agencies. Attacking these issues, however, is no more the responsibility of an IHCS than it is of other corporations in the area. Managed care plans should take the lead in having active programs in prevention and wellness, because they stand to reduce their own expenditures by keeping patients out of the hands of specialists and hospitals. If the IHCS does not have a managed care subsidiary but is only a provider of health care services, then the role of the IHCS is simply to encourage managed care plans operating in the local community to undertake such programs.

Reserved Rights Versus Local Autonomy

When IHCSs are formed, one of the first hurdles encountered is determining the extent to which local autonomy will be retained. By their very nature, alliances are generally unwilling to permit the organizing entity to have control over the decision making of the participating organizations. Since the decision to join is voluntary, the role of an alliance is greatly restricted and may be limited to securing managed care contracts that provide information and outcome results. In carrying out this role, the alliance may develop utilization guidelines for the participants. However, the scope of its activities is much narrower than that of more highly integrated health care systems.

In the case of a nonprofit hospital consolidating with another nonprofit hospital, both institutions may retain their governing boards even though a parent corporation board may be formed.

Systems run by Catholic orders tend to leave local governing boards in place. When a single hospital creates a parent organization, reserved rights typically are written into the bylaws. Reserved rights often restrict the subsidiary organizations in the appointment of board members, appointment of the chief executive, amendment of bylaws, approval of capital and operating budgets, sale of property, and dissolution or acquisition of debt; but because the formation of the IHCS occurs through voluntary agreements, the reserved rights are not enforced. Since the role of the parent organization is to coordinate activity, it most often does not have its own sources of revenue but is dependent upon assessing the subsidiaries for funds to cover its operations. Because of this dependent relationship, the parent organization becomes, in reality, a subsidiary of the subsidiaries and is in no position to enforce the reserved rights. Where a subsidiary is bought and paid for, the parent organization feels free to enforce reserved rights.

Collective Role of Physicians Versus Individual Autonomy

The most difficult challenge in the formation of a system is the integration of the physician component. The basic issue, however, that separates boards and management from physicians is not the control of the actual practice of medicine, which is and will remain a prerogative of physicians. Rather, the difficulty faced is a cultural issue. Physicians are trained to make definitive decisions and to act independently in diagnosing and treating patients. This habit spills over into the management of a practice. In both patient care and practice management, physicians are willing to seek advice and to refer patients to other physicians, but not to those outside the profession. As a result of this mind-set, physicians accustomed to making their own decisions have difficulty accepting organizational rules that inevitably are part of a large organization. Physicians who join large multispecialty group practices early in their professional careers do not develop the same habits, however, and are much more willing to acquiesce, since they are culturally conditioned to do so. For example, physicians joining the Kaiser-Permanente system or the Mayo Clinic system know that they will have to play by the system's rules. Simply by joining they are acknowledging a willingness to do so.

Forming a PHO as part of an IHCS in which the physicians are unaccustomed to being part of a larger whole leads to many unanticipated problems for both the PHO and the IHCS. Bringing about a cultural change among physician members is a long-term process that may interfere with the rate of development of the IHCS. This interference will be particularly evident in the thoughts expressed by physician board members. One of the real advantages of having physicians on the governing board is that they think about health care in terms of individuals, an orientation that counterbalances the approach of those who think in general terms. The thought process of physicians is from the particular to the general, while the thought process of executives is from the general to the particular. Both approaches are necessary in an IHCS, since the aim of an IHCS should be to achieve an optimal balance between the provision of acceptable care and the costs of that care. Striking such a balance is an ongoing struggle that will never be solved to everyone's satisfaction. Instead, it should be recognized that dynamic tension always will be part and parcel of the decision-making process of an IHCS.

Board Roles Versus Management Roles

The concept of hospital board involvement in health care systems has been considerably different from the concept of corporate board involvement. The differences are rooted in the fact that health care systems have developed from freestanding hospitals that were once charitable institutions whose board members served in a governance capacity because of their willingness and ability to cover any year-end losses. Because they were expected either to contribute funds to cover losses or to make major contributions to fund-raising activities, nonprofit hospital boards tended to view hospital managers as not being their equals as businesspersons. As a result of the financial responsibilities they accepted, board members saw themselves as community-minded citizens looking out for the welfare of the poor and the needy. Because of their commitment to charitable work, these boards decided who would become board members, what buildings would be built, and what new programs would be undertaken. It was a world uncomplicated by the complexities of today's health care environment.

While freestanding hospitals were metamorphosing into health care systems, corporate America was also undergoing its own transition. Individual entrepreneurs started up companies that would eventually become the giants of industry and whose governing boards became extensions of the chief executive. The role of the corporate board was to provide insight and to assist in bringing about the vision determined by the chief executive. Profits and financial viability were the keys to growth. As complexity increased, management expanded and took on an ever wider scope of activities. If other companies were bought, their governing boards simply disappeared as part of the transaction. Executives replaced governing boards. There would be no question of the board of the acquired company continuing to function, even if the corporation had multiple functions and multiple locations.

In large health care systems that have developed as for-profit enterprises, the board remains tied to economic considerations. It is in the nonprofit systems where confusion as to roles looms large. What prevails at the board meeting: community good or investor well-being? How do community concerns and interests get expressed if not through the involvement of local boards? Yet, what do such concerns contribute to the economic well-being of an IHCS that has a billion dollars or more of annual revenue, employees numbering in the thousands, and if not properly managed, an ability to have a profound negative impact on the communities in which its activities are carried out? How is a proper balance to be obtained and sustained in a health care environment that is undergoing rapid changes? Is it likely that as the IHCS grows it will take on more of a life of its own, that the needs of the organization will become so much larger and more important to those associated with the IHCS that the IHCS's relationship to the numerous local communities that health care services will fade into the background?

Among nonprofit integrated health care systems, board seats and the number of governing boards are often the medium of exchange, not dollars. The question, Are all of these boards necessary? is not addressed. If the answer is negative, the next question that arises is how to get rid of them. Can they be eliminated or must they be continued? In for-profit health care systems, excess boards are eliminated and replaced with advisory boards that lack organizational authority. But in nonprofit systems the typical structure retains governing boards. Why? The answer lies in the way IHCSs are built or established.

The question of whether to retain a governing board when one nonprofit entity joins with another nonprofit entity never arises. The only issue is whether to form a consolidated board or leave the boards separate. This type of decision is based on whether the acquired entity was purchased as an economic activity. If it was, the concern would be over the purchase price, not the board seats. When an entity is purchased, an economic transaction occurs; one party acquires the assets and liabilities of the second party. The second party receives either cash, shares, or a debt instrument, which ultimately converts to cash. Value has been exchanged, dollars have been received in exchange for an operational entity.

However, when two nonprofits enter into an agreement, no exchange of economic value takes place. The first party acquires decision-making authority over the second party, but the second party receives no economic value, even though it is now controlled. Since no tangible exchange has taken place, the only way of bringing about value for the acquired organization is to provide for board seats in the successor organization. Whether or not an additional board is actually useful, or whether or not an expanded board size is necessary, is not of concern at that point in time. All hands recognize that the governance issue is the key to bringing about a merger or consolidation, since money is not the medium of exchange. In order to join the two entities, the question about board size or numbers of boards is evaded and left to be resolved at some distant time in the future. Management is left with the problem of struggling to cope with the governance structure.

In time, an aggressive IHCS will consist of many boards and board members, which can reach as high as twenty boards with a total of two hundred or more board members. At such a point it becomes apparent to the key stakeholders that something needs to be done to alleviate the confusion that has built up in the process of creating the IHCS. Having avoided the purchase of entities and instead opted for alliances or consolidations, the disbanding of governing boards cannot be used as a remedy. Other measures have to be taken. Yet, at the same time, board members and management will recognize that finances have to be centralized. When seeking long-term debt or equity funds, investors are likely to insist on involving all of the related organization's assets. The key decision makers realize that in order to comply with this standard requirement for investments, the coordinating body for the IHCS needs to establish several reserved rights, which should include approval of budgets, capital expenditures beyond a given amount, sale or purchase of property, and changes in rate structure.

Typically left to the discretion of individual boards are fund-raising, credentialing of physicians, operational oversight, recommendations for new programs, and community development activities. Concurrence between the coordinating body and the individual entity is usually required for the employment of a new chief executive. When reserved rights are put in place and enforced, the role of the individual entity becomes one of looking out for the health care interests of the local community. In essence, it becomes the local health care watchdog. As long as local concerns are met, the coordinating body is free to expand, to undertake new activities, and to behave in a manner that satisfies the vision and objectives that it has determined meet the needs of the IHCS.

Since the enforcement of reserved rights is crucial to the success of the IHCS, the role of management expands to a considerable extent. Freed from having to answer to the plethora of governing boards, the IHCS takes on more of the characteristics of a for-profit organization, with the executives taking on more responsibilities, exercising greater authority, and being held accountable through the chain of command rather than to their respective governing boards.

In the process of developing these new relationships, the opportunities for misunderstandings to occur between the executives and the governing boards are increased considerably. Frequently, board members may believe that the chief executive officer and other executives have moved too far in front of governance and are undertaking tasks and projects before giving the board members sufficient time to review and approve what is going on. Slowing down the decision-making process to the speed with which the various governing boards can cope may not seem to be the appropriate thing for the executives to do as they assess what is going on in the marketplace. Under such circumstances, difficulties may arise between management and governance, which may result in the management being replaced.

Conclusions

The transition from an alliance of affiliates to an integrated health care system is likely to be the most difficult challenge facing nonprofit organizations. Simply providing for a variety of ways to interlock existing governing boards deals with symptoms, not underlying needs. If the desired end result is an integrated delivery system, the decision-making authority of multiple boards will be reduced significantly and the authority of management will be increased. In time, local government boards that are part of an IHCS will come to appreciate that their role is to be the advocate of local health care interests and to make enough noise to the parent organization so that their local interests are not neglected.

Part Four

Challenges for Managers and Physicians

Chapter Sixteen

The Metamorphosis of a Hospital Chief Executive

Richard L. Johnson

The ideas presented in this chapter about the metamorphosis of a hospital chief executive may lead the reader to conclude that I wholeheartedly endorse the changes that are now under way in the health care field. Such is not the case. What I discuss here is what I *believe* will take place, but it is not what I would *prefer* to have happen. The trends now in motion will lead to these results, but in doing so, many of the values that have made American medicine and hospitals the envy of the world will be lost. For the losses, I am profoundly sad.

The intense competition that now places economic results above medical care has resulted in a health care climate dominated by fear. In the environment now emerging, CEO careers will be made and broken in relatively short periods of time. Bruising battles will be fought in the competitive arena, and attention to detail will be a day-to-day fight that will go on with no end in sight. Kindness and gentleness will not be values held in high regard. What will count will be the ability to produce the desired financial results through productivity and quality improvements. This is the formula for success required when economics dominates the health care environment.

Building on the Past

By the time a professionally-trained health care executive reaches the position of chief executive of a hospital, he or she is typically in the forty-plus age range. In the majority of cases, the person has obtained a graduate degree in health care management. Some have served for a number of years in administrative roles in a variety of hospitals, moving over time into positions of increasing responsibility. Others with the same educational background have remained in one hospital but have progressed from one position to another while gaining experience and responsibility. Finally, the opportunity arises and the individual moves into the top position of president and chief executive officer (CEO). What kinds of baggage does this person bring along as a result of having spent fifteen to twenty years working his or her way to the top?

Over those years, the second- or third-level executive had daily contact with the chief executive, and from time to time would attend meetings of the governing board as matters under the executive's control were discussed. In the course of daily activities, the second- or third-level executive inevitably would form opinions about how the chief executive handled the board and treated internal operational activities. In the process, the second- or third-level executive would form opinions about how he or she would act when in the position of CEO.

By the time the executive arrived at the top, he or she had developed his or her own behavior patterns. In a sense, each CEO is a composite picture of his or her personal and professional experiences. Without consciously thinking about it, each CEO decides which reports that cross his or her desk are important, how much time to spend on board matters, what community activities are of interest, how involved to become in medical staff affairs—all of which ultimately fit into a pattern of priorities. In many respects, CEOs become captives of their own previous experiences. In their mind's eye they have an image of what they see as the role of the hospital within the spectrum of health care services and programs. However, CEOs are now confronted with realities that are forcing hospitals into new roles as they struggle to deal with PHOs, affiliations, business coalitions, capitation plans, managed care, and integrated delivery systems. Increasingly, CEOs are facing new dimensions in health care for which their education and experience do not provide any guidance for the future.

Determining the Future

Given the uncertainties that now surround the role of hospital chief executives, they often find themselves asking themselves such questions as the following:

- Should the hospital affiliate with a larger hospital?
- Should the hospital become part of a university medical center?
- Should the hospital become the leading health care system in its region of the state?
- What does the adjusted cost per patient day have to be in order for the hospital to successfully bid on managed care contracts?
- To what extent can the hospital develop into a successful PHO?
- Can the hospital afford to increase its long-term debt in order to remain on the cutting edge of medical technology?
- What will it cost the hospital to recruit primary care physicians and how can their permanence be assured if recruitment efforts are successful?
- Will Medicare and Medicaid become part of managed care and will the hospital be forced into bidding on these contracts?
- How many beds will the hospital need to operate in the years ahead as utilization rates continue downward?
- How can the hospital's survival be ensured as conditions change?

The president of the hospital has a sense of responsibility about determining the future direction of the organization. Recognizing that "business as usual" will no longer be a satisfactory course to follow, the CEO is aware that the role of leadership requires selecting a new route. Hospital CEOs instinctively appreciate that their governing boards look to them for direction. Individual board members may have their own ideas, but they are most likely to take direction from their president on this important matter, based on their belief that the CEO is more in tune with what is going on in the health care field.

Determining the future course of a hospital requires evaluating a complex set of conditions that will have varying impacts on the organization. Since many of these factors are in the early stages of development, CEOs recognize that the chances of making mistakes may be substantial. Not only do presidents need to consider the speed with which new trends may develop, but they have to evaluate the internal support or disagreement that may ensue. The variables that must be considered include the following:

- The growth rate of managed care and capitation in the community
- The competitive environment in which the hospital finds itself
- The attitude of medical staff members about forming an integrated delivery system with the hospital
- The financial condition of the hospital
- The governing board's willingness to give up some of its autonomy, if needed

Sorting out these factors is a difficult task because it involves estimating the reactions of the various groups of stakeholders to what may be proposed, knowing that changes in trends in the external environment will also lead to shifts in opinions among the stakeholders. CEOs find themselves confronted with two types of decisions: those related to the course the hospital should follow, and those related to how support is to be obtained from among the decision makers and influence makers.

Given the degree of uncertainty about the future and the necessity for gaining support for any decisions reached, some CEOs will put off dealing with the new realities as long as possible and limit their role to responding to the hospital's day-to-day activities. They will not attempt to fashion a plan for the future that encompasses programs and activities that lie outside the traditional domain of the hospital. Nevertheless, even though the CEOs' focus will remain traditional, they will appreciate that the following changes will occur:

- The annual number of inpatient days of care will continue to erode slowly from one year to the next.
- Medicare patient days will continue to rise slowly from one year to the next.

- Patient revenues from commercial indemnity insurance will gradually disappear as a source of income.
- The number of full-time employees needed will decline and additional layoffs will be necessary.
- The need to increase productivity will have to be a major concern of management.
- The growth rate of hospital outpatient services will slow down as physicians provide more and more ambulatory services in their offices.
- The number of lives covered by managed care plans will continue to grow.
- The net profit margin of the hospital will probably decline from one year to the next.

The kind of thinking that will be required to make the transition is a reversal of past patterns, in which the prevailing approach was to continually shore up the internal operations and expand the comprehensiveness of the services offered. The belief that guided the provision of hospital care for many decades was "the best possible care at the lowest possible cost." Looked at in light of the growth and support of managed care concepts in this country, this belief is no longer viable. It was based on an individual hospital doing what was needed to become a technological institution, a concern with internal operations.

With the growing dominance in managed care, this is an inappropriate strategy. The reverse is now needed. Instead of an orientation of being on the inside looking out, what is now required is an orientation of being on the outside looking in, which requires an understanding of marketplace forces. Market pressures are now strong enough to bring about changes in the health care scene. It is no longer a matter of simply responding to the health care needs of a primary service area, but a question of how large a health care system is needed to command a market presence in a particular region so that all of the other players will have to recognize the necessity for dealing with the system. Instead of thinking in terms of a marketplace within a five-mile radius of the hospital, market presence may have to be considered within a radius of eighty to one hundred miles. The outside-in approach requires far more than locating a few primary care centers to function as a network for feeding patients to the sponsoring hospital. Rather, this approach is based on ultimately owning a substantial part, if not all, of the revenue stream of a per-member, per-month managed care plan encompassing a large area.

Being aware that these changes are likely to take place leads a CEO to have an uneasy feeling that steps should be taken to position the hospital so that it will survive and continue to operate. What is needed to make this happen is a metamorphosis from traditional thinking to new patterns of thought. The CEO's work habits developed over years need to be discarded and replaced with new habits. The traditional role of being the internal manager of operations has in most hospitals already been shifted to another person, such as a second-level executive, who has become the lightning rod for handling all of the operational problems that arise on a daily basis. The behaviors of internal departmental managers must be modified by the understanding that the CEO is no longer available to deal with their problems. This is often a difficult transition for both departmental managers and the CEO. Departmental managers may see such a shift in responsibility as a downgrading of their own positions and may therefore ignore it and continue to report to the top. At the same time, the CEO may be reluctant to enforce the new organizational alignment because it means giving up the relationships, reports, and responsibilities that are most familiar. In the back of the CEO's mind will always be the thought that whatever new program or activity is started, the basic reason for it should be to improve results, as well as to stabilize the level and mix of patient revenues. A continuing effort has to be made to avoid falling back into a comfortable routine.

Moving into new territory leads to increased concern about what the future holds. This concern is shared by physicians, who are anxious about retaining practice revenues at existing levels. Many physicians are fearful that the anticipated growth of managed care will result in maintaining existing work levels but for lower levels of revenue. Fears about the future may lead to heightened tensions within the hospital organization as each participant strives to protect his or her own economic turf.

CEOs will discover that the decisions they need to make no longer fall within the scope of authority they have had in the past, but to go beyond the scope is to abandon a traditional role, which many CEOs see as taking enormous personal risks. The CEO's role and experiences of the past become a cage that acts as a deterrent to change. The CEO not only has to escape from the past, but at the same time he or she must begin to shift board members and physician leaders' perceptions into new ways of looking at the future. This is never an easy task, but it may be particularly difficult to accomplish if the governing board has come to view the CEO as an operations manager rather than as a competent executive accustomed to a leadership role.

In those hospitals where the CEO views his or her role as being an operations manager, or where the governing board views the CEO as an operations manager, the future of the hospital is predictable. The downward spiral of organizational trends will continue until there is widespread acceptance among the key stakeholders that the future holds bankruptcy unless drastic action is taken, at which point consideration may be given to becoming part of a health care system and giving up ownership of the hospital.

New Reference Points

Recognizing that such an outcome is a possibility creates a sense of urgency in the CEO to be willing to explore new opportunities, even at the risk of personal difficulties, or organizational failure. To deal with the emerging realities, a CEO needs to develop a frame of reference that is not based on filling inpatient beds but rather is concerned primarily with capturing as much managed care revenue as possible. This means that the emphasis must shift away from spending funds on building new facilities or remodeling old ones, because the acute care hospital will no longer be the centerpiece of health care. What is needed is a system in which appropriate health services can be obtained in a reasonable, convenient manner in decentralized settings. A balance must be maintained between centralized decision making and individual-unit autonomy, and this need has to be recognized throughout the hospital in both revenue and expense determinations. This type of organization requires a sophisticated information infrastructure for financial, clinical, and administrative data, and reports need to link all of the units together. The driving force is decentralized decision making but centralized coordination.

This approach requires a chief executive to devote primary attention to thinking strategically, a different mind-set from what is needed for overseeing the daily operations of a hospital. To undertake the metamorphosis is a challenging assignment because it means that the chief executive has to, on his or her own initiative, stop spending time on those activities that were part and parcel of his or her former role. Time can no longer be spent reactively dealing with matters in short spurts and issuing orders in response to the immediate problems confronting second- and third-level executives. The chief executive needs to rearrange his or her commitments so that major chunks of time are available for planning, studying, and negotiating with others, all of which must be accomplished in an internal environment that has been accustomed to a very different behavior pattern on the part of the chief executive. Not only does the chief executive have to change his or her own behavior, but the behavior of those around the chief executive has to be modified as well if the end result is to be a health care system, not just a hospital.

When confronted with the necessity for making the shift to a strategic mode, the chief executive may be tempted to insert a chief operating officer into the organizational structure in order to free up the needed time from his or her own schedule for strategic planning and negotiations. Such a move may fail if the sole consideration is need. The timing can be important; making such a move has to be carefully considered and given sufficient attention. Before such a step can be successfully implemented, the governing board, second- and third-level executives, and leadership of the medical staff have to reach the point of understanding and accepting such a move as being in the best interests of the organization. If the move to insert a chief operating officer occurs precipitously, the desired results may not be accomplished. Instead of encountering a receptive climate for such a change, the insertion of a chief operating officer may be read negatively by the governing board, second- and third-level executives, and medical staff leadership as a ploy on the part of the chief executive to avoid dealing with the "real" problems of the hospital. Should such an opinion become widespread among these various groups, the end result is predictable: the chief executive will be replaced.

The lesson to be learned is that these three groups have to accept the necessity for the chief executive to move into the strategic role before such a move can be implemented. Once this understanding has been accomplished, the shift can be made. What remains is the question of whether the chief executive can succeed in transforming the hospital into a health care system.

Different Skills Needed

In making the transition from the traditional hospital role to the new role, the CEO is confronted with two different but closely related personal issues: What skills have to be learned? and Where does one find the time to learn these new skills? The sets of skills needed to lead an organization strategically are different from those skills needed to manage it. Bringing strategic skills into focus after spending fifteen to twenty years using managerial skills is not an easy assignment. To accomplish such a task the CEO must first decide whether it is a necessity, and then he or she must undertake a self-taught course in loosening the managerial ties, practiced in his or her day-to-day activities, while at the same time beginning to move in the direction of strategic activities. An inner compass is needed to guide this development over time.

A Sense of Direction

In order to transform a hospital into a health care system, the CEO has to have a clear sense of where he or she wants to take the organization. At every opportunity, other stakeholders should be reminded of the new direction. Repeating the new direction over and over again ultimately builds support because the theme is consistent. The CEO comes to be regarded as one who intends to see the process through to completion and who is not likely to stop short of the goals established. Such comments as "You'd better get aboard the train if you don't want to be run over by the locomotive" will be heard occasionally within the organization. This type of statement reflects that the message is getting through to the stakeholders.

Negotiation Skills

One of the most important attributes of a CEO who is endeavoring to build a strategic organization is the ability to deal with uncertainty. Since strategic relationships may involve contracting with other health care providers, negotiation skills are an important tool. To successfully use them, the CEO has to be patient and a good listener, so that mutually agreed upon positions are worked out step by step. As part of this process, the CEO has to come across to the other party in negotiations as open and honest, so that a bridge of trust is developed. While the CEO will want to convey a sense of urgency about completing negotiations, it must be handled in such a way that the CEO does not come across as being impatient.

Decision-Making Authority

One of the more difficult tasks is to learn what decisions must be made on one's own authority. When negotiations are undertaken, there often arises an occasion when a CEO clearly recognizes that a decision on his or her part is required immediately if the process is to be successfully concluded. When this happens, the CEO cannot halt the negotiating process but has to make a decision right then and there, and he or she cannot refer it to the governing board for approval before the next steps can be taken. To defer a decision to a later date in order to get the necessary approval signals to the other parties in the negotiations that they are dealing with an individual who lacks the necessary authority. This suggests that negotiations are going on at the wrong organizational level. Yet, if the CEO goes ahead and commits the hospital without consulting the board, he or she runs the risk of being accused of exceeding his or her authority.

This type of dilemma will arise with increasing frequency as a hospital takes on an expanded role with physician organizations, managed care plans, and other health care providers. Commitments for the expenditure of hundreds of thousands of dollars may have to be made on such short notice that it is impractical to convene a meeting of the governing board in order to get their approval of the expenditure. An alternative is to inform the governing board of this potential challenge and to get their authority to step beyond what has been delegated when it is in the best interests of the organization. The dynamics of the current health care environment are dictating rapid decision making and far more flexibility of authority than traditionally exercised by community hospital CEOs. As hospitals form into larger and larger groupings of health care providers, governing boards will have less and less control over the economics of the organization. Revenues will be dictated by the terms of managed care contracts, while large capital expenditures will be determined as a result of negotiations with other parties to an affiliation. This will leave little or no room for governing board involvement, except for after-the-fact support.

In addition, a CEO has to deal with his or her ego. Having reached a point in his or her career where a high degree of self-confidence is mandatory, having to give up the right to make decisions across the board and to accept the fact that final authority may be vested in someone else makes the voluntary relinquishing of authority a major hurdle. The same type of problem also faces the members of a governing board if they decide to merge with another hospital or health system. For this reason, affiliations have appealed to many CEOs and governing boards, because in an affiliation the individual hospital boards do not have to give up any authority.

Entrepreneurial Skills

For health care systems to have decentralized service points but centralized coordination requires not only a sophisticated information system but also a mechanism for funneling funds within the system. If the hospital has an ownership interest in the managed care plan, it benefits through its share of the net profits. Without such ownership, the hospital has to rely on developing a system of physicians and outlying hospitals that will refer tertiary care patients, thereby bolstering patient services.

To develop a system that can provide care at diverse points in the marketplace, a CEO has to hone entrepreneurial skills, which are very different from managerial skills. Rather than thinking in terms of fixed costs, a CEO has to view the majority of operating costs as variables so that maximum productivity is achieved. Much of what goes on in a hospital is thought of in terms of fixed revenues and fixed expenses. Decisions are made by comparing the two and then deciding to adjust the overall budget in order to achieve the desired results. But in a managed care environment with diverse points of service, administrative judgments have to be made on an incremental basis, one at a time. Fine-tuning of the system requires detailed planning, not global judgments.

In this new setting, the chief executive has to see to it that the information reviewed contains a detailed analysis of what is needed. Large group meetings have to be replaced with small, highly specialized, focused meetings that always have a sense of urgency about them. The attention of the CEO has to shift from serving the governing board's interests to focusing on the major concern of dealing with the broad spectrum of health care issues in the marketplace. Internal operations no longer dominate the CEO's agenda; they are replaced with concerns about managed care contracts, physician participation, percentage of marketplace penetration, increased productivity, dealing with business coalitions, and other assorted external factors.

Creating a New Climate

Creating a climate for strategic planning and negotiating requires large amounts of uninterrupted time so that issues can be explored thoroughly. The need for this time may not be fully appreciated by a CEO who has spent years dealing with problems in short time frames. Relearning is required when one has to stop responding to immediate demands on one's time. Even though CEOs had removed themselves as line managers when they realized they had to concentrate on strategic issues, they had to continually exercise responsibility for following up on their own projects. This experience may turn out to be a stumbling block to a CEO accustomed to having a large staff of administrative personnel to whom to delegate managerial problems, because the support staff for strategic planning is usually very limited in number or composed of line managers who are expected to devote only part of their time to strategic planning. It usually turns out that line duties are viewed as more important than strategic projects because of the immediacy of the problems encountered. As a result, expectations of how much time is to be spent on strategic issues are never met. Follow-through depends primarily on the chief executive. Since strategic projects (such as creating PHOs or establishing alliances) usually require weeks, months, or even years to reach completion, it is important that they be monitored all the way along and that interest in them be maintained over the entire cycle. When there are unanticipated intervening problems, they must be dealt with before progress can be resumed. This requires tenaciousness on the part of the CEO.

In the emerging integrated delivery system, the role of physicians will be increasingly important. Physicians are significant partners, even though their orientation is considerably different than that of the CEO. The greater the CEO's understanding of the values physicians hold dear, and the more clinical knowledge he or she has gained in previous experiences in hospital management, the greater will be the trust that can be established when negotiations are undertaken in developing a health care system with physicians.

Fundamental to successful negotiations for the CEO is an appreciation of the degree of patience and fortitude required. Internal turmoil often occurs as a negotiating process unfolds. The CEO's role is particularly difficult in that he or she may well be viewed as holding all of the financial cards, and he or she may be expected to use some of the accumulated cash reserves of the hospital to underwrite whatever costs are incurred for developing the PHO.

The Attractiveness of Affiliations

Rather than face up to the difficulties of creating a health care system, the hospital may desire to take a more limited step by turning to affiliation. The rationale for doing so is a desire to stay uncommitted and see what happens. This frame of mind implies that marketplace pressures are not yet strong enough to lead to more closely tied relationships. If the CEO reaches this conclusion, then an alternative course of action, such as affiliating with a larger hospital or a university medical center, is viewed as a way of remaining a player in the managed care environment. The efforts to win managed care contracts appear to improve under such arrangements.

The affiliation is attractive because it leaves intact the autonomy of the hospital. It is a voluntary arrangement that does not involve the consolidation of assets and liabilities, and it therefore appeals to both the CEO and members of the governing board. No organizational authority is taken away; instead, such an arrangement is based on the belief that an affiliation forces managed care plans to recognize that they have to contract with the affiliated parties. Typically, hospitals that join an affiliation fail to recognize sufficiently how this strategy affects the planning of a managed care company. If the affiliation is viewed by the managed care plan executives as a stumbling block to what they are trying to accomplish, they will attempt to split off selected members of the affiliation by suggesting shifts to increase the volume of services to one hospital. In return, they may expect a lower price per unit of service. This type of offer is based on the expectation that it will lead to the crumbling of the voluntary affiliation. Without stringent contract provisions among the affiliates that provide penalties for leaving the affiliation, the strategy of splitting apart the group may just turn out to be successful.

Another alternative that has been tried is the development of local, vertically integrated health care systems. These are "seamless" organizations in which the hospital controls home health, durable medical equipment, ambulatory surgery sites, primary care locations, and nursing homes, all in the local area. To date, this approach has not demonstrated an ability to withstand the marketplace pressures that can be exerted by managed care plans.

Changing the Focus

By and large, most hospital CEOs recognize that having the most comprehensive range of acute diagnostic and therapeutic services no longer commands the support it once engendered. CEOs are fully aware that economics has become the gatekeeper of the health care system. Managed care plans are recognized as "owning" blocks of patients, and in order to be successful in dealing with managed care plans, a hospital has to be aware that its chances of winning provider contracts are enhanced if the hospital has the following characteristics:

- It is a low-cost provider of acute services.
- It has a good reputation in the community.
- Its service area is large.

- It has an ongoing program of measuring clinical outcomes.
- It has integrated its delivery system with physicians.
- It controls a "seamless" system so that patients are treated at the appropriate level of care.

In the competitive arena that now pervades the health care field, the ability to put the pieces of a health care system into place in a relatively short period may be of prime importance. If speed is of concern, relying on debt money for capital expenditures may not be sufficient. Resorting to loans and accumulated reserves of cash as the sole sources of expansion may turn out to be too limiting in the face of vigorous competition from for-profit entities. Hospital CEOs need to appreciate that competition is no longer from just other nonprofit hospitals, but may be from for-profit hospital systems, managed care plans, or insurance carriers with deep pockets who are willing to spend ten to twenty times as much for accomplishing their goals in the same market area. When such circumstances arise, the playing field is no longer level and the losers are the nonprofit hospitals that cannot match the speed or spending power of the for-profit entities that have elected to enter the marketplace. To counter this type of activity, CEOs need to adopt strategies that do not involve spending large amounts of money to purchase other health care providers; instead, they need to develop strong contractual relationships among the affiliates.

Where health care activities take place is an important consideration in developing a strategic plan. Hospital CEOs tend to view patient care in terms of a hub and spokes, where the hospital is the hub and physician offices are the spokes. Such a viewpoint is not a viable concept in a managed care environment. Rather, the concept has to envision patient care occurring at any number of sites, including other hospitals, nursing homes, physicians' offices, and home health agencies—wherever the appropriate level of service can be provided in a manner that is reasonably convenient to patients.

Survival Rates

Looking to the future, the question may be asked, What will be the survival rate of CEOs? Two approaches may be taken in looking at the future. Certainly the age of a CEO will have an impact. Those who have been CEOs for a number of years and are probably a decade or less away from retirement are likely to continue in the same mode as they have in the past. Those at the other end of the age spectrum, who have just become CEOs, are likely to adopt new patterns of behavior that reflect the changing conditions under which CEOs are going to have to perform. Those CEOs who are in-between the two extremes of age may or may not change. To some extent, the need to change depends on the size of the community in which the hospital is located.

The second approach depends not on age but on the size of the community and the amount of managed care in it. Large metropolitan cities are the most likely to have substantial percentages of managed care, fierce competition among hospitals, and rapid development of health systems. The name of the game is most likely to be "swallow" your neighboring hospital or be swallowed by the other hospital. Eventually, only three or four health care systems will survive.

In small towns and villages, managed care will arrive much later than it has in cities, after the major markets have been saturated by managed care companies. When managed care does arrive, the traditional hospital will either be absorbed into a health care system or it is likely to see a steadily declining census and ultimately go out of business.

In midsize communities, where there may be three to six hospitals, the short-run outcomes are difficult to predict. Some CEOs will become aggressive and attempt to develop local systems of health care. Success will come to some, and failure to others. Experience seems to indicate that more will fail than will succeed in making the metamorphosis to a new role.

Conclusions

If, as seems likely, the growth of hospitals into larger and larger health care corporations comes about, the need for capital funds will increase and outstrip the system's ability to rely on debt financing and the use of savings. To continue to grow, consideration will have to be given to the use of equity financing and there may be widespread development of for-profit organizations. The likelihood of becoming for-profit will be in keeping with the typical development of integrated systems of hospitals and physicians. Physicians typically prefer a for-profit corporate form because it offers an opportunity to share in any profits that might result. If the movement of hospitals into for-profit health care systems comes about, it will be due to the pressures created by the need for equity funds and by the increasingly important role of physicians in integrated delivery systems.

Once equity funds and long-term debt become a substantial part of the financing of health care systems, CEOs will be faced with having to deal with the values of Wall Street rather than Main Street. To their dismay, CEOs will discover that they are confronted with investor expectations that are far different from the expectations the CEOs hold dear. Rather than focusing on programs that will provide better health for all of the people in the community and that will require long time frames to accomplish and result in minimal financial returns, CEOs will find that they are expected to produce profits that are measured on a quarterly or annual basis. It will become apparent that the time line between actual operational results and budget expectations is only thirty to ninety days. The name of the game becomes achieving financial results acceptable to both equity and debt investors, not doing good for the community. An emphasis on quality of care, a focus on comprehensiveness of up-to-date technology, and a desire to care for those unable to pay in the face of less-than-expected profit margins are viewed as excuses for poor financial results. CEOs who cling to these notions will have short careers. The traditional values associated with nonprofit hospitals and health care systems will inevitably become secondary to the primary interest of obtaining an acceptable rate of return on investment. If both ends can be accomplished, the best of both worlds will have been achieved.

The degree of pressure on CEOs to practice as economically as possible is much greater than the pressure on physicians. Physicians have long recognized the desirability of controlling every dollar of expense in the management of their practices since their own incomes decline if they fail to do so. Conversely, physicians have expected the hospitals to provide all of the necessary resources that enable them to diagnose and treat patients at a level that satisfies the physicians' professional sense of what is needed.

This expectation places the CEO of a for-profit hospital in the unenviable position of having to satisfy two masters, the practitioner and the investor. If the resources to do both become constrained, difficult choices have to be made.

A second type of pressure has now emerged. Employers are taking harder and harder looks at their expenditures for health care benefits for their employees. Many employers are now in world markets and in order to survive in highly competitive arenas they have had to improve the quality of their products while at the same time reducing prices. Having learned that lesson, they have similar expectations as purchasers of health care. Their view of the health care marketplace is that it is highly competitive and that they can take advantage of it in order to reduce their expenditures for health care and to provide greater convenience for their employees. Hospitals should respond to this employer expectation by providing them with detailed reports on how they have decreased hospital costs through increased productivity and by working with physicians to adopt clinical protocols and clinical outcomes that reduce patient costs.

In addition, hospitals, outpatient facilities, physician offices—in fact, all providers—are going to have to become much more patient-friendly. Physicians who continue to expect patients to wait for an hour or more to be seen for a fifteen-minute scheduled appointment, or clinics who have patients waiting for two or three hours for a procedure that lasts a few minutes, will find that this waiting is no longer acceptable. Health care providers who are successful in the years ahead will stress patient convenience, carefully developed clinical protocols based on outcome measures, and statistics that clearly demonstrate quality improvements and lower costs to the payer of the bill for services.

Learning these lessons is a difficult challenge for both physicians and CEOs. Putting them into practice day after day requires major adjustments in attitudes and behavior patterns, along with a willingness to change. Leadership in health care organizations will belong to those CEOs who are able to make the transition. The question to be resolved is whether the caterpillar will become a butterfly or the butterfly become a caterpillar.

Chapter Seventeen

Physician Opportunities in Management

Signs and Portents

Montague Brown

In the 1960s, organizational theory and the sociology of professions indicated that there was strong evidence that whenever professions were brought into bureaucracies, members of the profession attempted to take over control of the management of the profession. There is evidence of this in the medical service branches of the military. Engineers in business seek dual degrees, as well as promotion into the ranks of management, as do scientists in other disciplines. Dual tracks often exist, making it necessary more often than not for professionals in large bureaucracies to shift into management in order to further their economic reward path. Unions of professionals often complement this individual effort to exert control over the profession.

During the past ten years, there has been an explosion of change that has brought physicians increasingly under the control of organizations, and this shift should present opportunities for physicians in management.

Note: A version of this chapter was published using the same title in *Physician Executive,* December 1994, *20,* pp. 3–8. Used here with permission of American College of Physician Executives.

Positive Trends

Shift from Not-for-Profit Institutions to Market Equity Models

Major change is occurring in the ownership and control of physician practices, community and university hospitals, and managed care companies.[1] These changes are offering physicians an opportunity to own equity shares in community hospitals, in managed care companies, in networks, and in their own practices, once they sell out to other entities. These are not merely locally owned businesses; they are frequently market equity firms whose stock is traded daily on national exchanges.

As these ventures emerge, physicians in coordinating, managing, and leadership roles have substantial opportunities to take on management roles and ownership roles. A postulate of the debate I have had with Richard Johnson and others is that physicians can own and operate some of these for-profit businesses during a critical transition period from the entrepreneurial start-up phase until the firm is of sufficient size, scope, and profitability that it needs heavy capital infusion to grow and/or until the physician owners want to convert their ownership interest into stock that has a ready market, so that they can cash out at will. When physicians own such organizations,[2] they have great opportunities to gain stature as managers and to have substantial roles. Indeed, some physicians will not only grow in managerial and executive stature, but they will also own substantial shares in the new firms, making it possible and desirable for them to take on major executive and governance roles when their firms go public or are sold to public firms.

Vertical Integration

No subject is hotter today than the concept of vertical integration. For many, this term means the merging or melding of physician practices and hospital organizations. Sometimes physicians acquire hospitals; sometimes the process is reversed. There is also an element of integration with physicians building and operating managed care firms, and integration occurs when insurers and managed care firms acquire and operate physician practices within their managed care operations.

Changes in Blue Cross and Blue Shield

Just as there are changes taking place in the ownership and operation of hospitals and medical practices, there also are major shifts going on in the Blue Cross and Blue Shield companies. These firms seek to recapture market share and roles from managed care firms that have done an end run on the more traditional Blue Cross/Blue Shield plans. They are also looking to acquire physician practices, especially primary care, and hospitals. Some are joint venturing with hospitals and physician groups.

Teaching Hospitals and Health Science Centers

There have always been opportunities for physicians in management, coordination, and executive roles in and around academic institutions. A solid research and teaching career often lays the groundwork for selection into the ranks of executive leadership.

Something new is happening, however, as vertical integration trends emerge. Distinguished institutions such as Emory University and the Medical University of South Carolina are teaming up with Columbia/HCA to form major joint ventures to own and operate hospitals and networks of primary care practices. As these hybrid organizations emerge, they will have physicians in major leadership roles. If community hospitals need medical directors, university hospitals and their faculty practice plans will expect no less, and probably more.

In these examples, the management of the physician practice groups falls to the university side of the business. One can also reasonably expect Columbia/HCA to sprout some new roles for physicians in the process. Teaching institutions have always been fertile ground for physicians who want to move into management, but today those opportunities are expanding as other systemic changes occur.

Payment Trends

Changes in payment methodologies have made it increasingly important for hospitals to work much more closely with medical staffs. With diagnosis-related groups, hospitals needed the understanding, support, and active involvement of medical staffs to bring utilization patterns in line with reimbursement. The economic incentives for physicians have been insufficient to make this happen. Whenever hospitals need to reach out to physicians, they tend to go through the elected leadership, but they must increasingly utilize full-time medical directors to keep closer ties on a regular and full-time basis.

Medical directors and full-time chiefs have long been noted for helping to bring to hospitals a degree of order and focus on quality outcomes and process. However, it has been the revolution in payment mechanisms that has brought about greater pressure to have full-time physicians working closely with the medical staff. Anyone working in such roles has ample opportunities to observe, learn about, and emulate executive behaviors. Equally important, they have positions that can be used to justify participation, at institutional expense, in management development activities. This is a traditional route to larger preparation, which is itself a route to better jobs in the management arena.

Of course, physicians taking on such roles must make choices about how they approach the roles. Some wear white coats and participate in meetings with a view toward expressing the physician's view. Others try to maintain their physician perspective and keep close tabs on where physician opinion lies, but they also try to participate in management meetings as managers, with a clear eye on institutional and management objectives. No doubt there are others who become such a management fixture that the original role of physician liaison is neglected. To grow and prosper in management means increasingly taking on the management role, building expertise in management, and becoming more and better known as an executive who also has empathy for and insight into medical needs in institutions.

Managed Care

With the advent of managed care, it has become even more important for all health care professionals to have detailed understanding of costs and processes that drive costs. Managed care brings new management opportunities for physicians. One psychiatrist friend tells me that he has stopped practicing and now makes a good living handling the review-and-expert role for a managed care company.

Marketing and professional relations create other opportunities. In staff-model plans, becoming the CEO is a good prospect for the physician who has the political, policy, and executive skills necessary for the role. Being a physician helps here, but it is no guarantee, even in physician-owned managed care companies.

Managed care also brings new opportunities for physicians associated with hospitals. Keeping track of costs, care maps, and protocols and finding ways to improve economic and quality performance in caring for patients are high on many agendas. Physicians have an edge in this arena.

There will be additional opportunities in general management for physicians who seek broader roles. Excellent roles exist in large corporations that want their own internal expertise in managed care. Managed care firms and divisions need managers; having an executive who has both medical and management expertise is a bonus.

Beyond a career in managed care, many opportunities exist for physicians with managed care expertise who want to move back into hospitals, group practices, and other more-integrated organizations. Just as lawyers often take apprentice roles as prosecutors, tax enforcers, and the like, so too can physicians learn and develop the art and craft of management and then return to more interesting and higher-level roles in organizations that they have learned about from the outside.

Cost Containment

As more and more employers and managed care buyers seek hard evidence of quality and cost-effectiveness, increasing attention will be given to quality process tools and techniques. Physicians with an interest and training in measurement techniques, process interaction, and engineering types of skills will have ample opportunity to play leadership roles in such hospital teams and in departments pursuing quality-of-care issues. Of course, there will also be people trained specifically in tools and techniques (statisticians) who will be competitors for such jobs, but the prepared physician has added value.

Outside of those organizations directly involved in providing care and measuring their results, there are many entrepreneurial opportunities for physicians who want to supply services but not work for established organizations. Develop a new measurement tool. Develop a company that does surveys and then sells data analysis to those who need to use it. Go into the training business and teach people how to do it. Join a policing outfit, learn their tools and techniques, and then develop a consulting practice to help people and organizations routinely look good according to the measures and methods being used to police the industry.

There are simply thousands of opportunities here. Some are managerial, some entrepreneurial, some policy-related, and many are a mix of all three. In a profession increasingly policed by outsiders, policing jobs abound.

Group Practice Development

Group practices will continue to develop and grow in size and complexity. This means greater opportunities for managers. Physicians have a natural opportunity to play leadership roles in such organizations, but for those who aspire to long-term leadership and management roles, there should be a continued quest for in-depth management training and experience, especially in areas of finance and health policy.

In smaller groups and primary care clusters put together on behalf of hospitals, there will be opportunities for physicians to get a taste of management roles by taking on leadership roles. Having a lead role in such clusters provides physicians with the opportunity both to exercise internal management skills and to negotiate among contiguous groups and entities.

PPOs and PHOs

Helping to build networks and joint venture operations can open up many opportunities in management. With an increasing trend toward vertical integration, some networks will become very large and complex operations. In fact, it is highly likely that some of these organizations will become giants that swallow hospitals, management care organizations, physician practices, and insurers.

These organizations are at the intersection of physician and hospital resources. There is leverage at these intersections for physicians to use in getting a better deal for practicing physicians. Whenever it is possible to exert leverage for the benefit of large groups and institutions, the roles that dominate such organizations tend to be those from which institutional leaders are selected.

Negative Trends

Most of the trends just considered could be subsumed under payment changes and integration. The list of changes could be expanded, and anyone with a fertile imagination could come up with dozens of opportunities that result from each change. However, there are some downsides or countertrends to consider.

Long-Term Trend to Institutional Ownership of Medical Practice

If current trends continue, it seems likely that most medicine will be practiced in some form of organization. Physicians will be employees and will have some major roles in the management of their colleagues.

Some physicians will have opportunities during the transition years to own equity interest in the emerging new organizations and thus play roles more akin to entrepreneurship than to institutional management. Young physicians entering practice today will never be able to develop an independent practice, and thus may never have an opportunity to convert a private practice into a business that can be sold. Managerial opportunities will become more the norm for upward mobility for practicing physicians, in organizations owned by others.

Professional Managers

If the world of professional managers is any guide to the future, there are plenty of competitors for physicians as they seek major roles in the management of health care organizations. This trend is best exemplified by the comments of one executive with a health administration degree who said, "What do you mean we need to get more physicians into management? Those guys already have too much power, and besides, this is our turf. We should not be giving them more." (For several reasons, I do not identify this person; but

I might add that this person was married to a physician! I do not think that being married to a physician influenced the comment, because I have found many others willing to voice such sentiments. No doubt, an experienced physician with substantial executive credentials is a major threat to many managers.) Physicians seeking to break into the executive ranks need to cultivate friends and colleagues who will help with mentorship, education, and experiential learning. Not everyone will be willing, but many will.

Independent Institutions in Placid Times Versus Cutthroat Competition

In the golden days of hospital administration, each chief executive officer had a board to report to and a medical staff to keep happy. Reimbursement was cost-plus, and most problems could be resolved by throwing money at them. Today's job is tougher and more complex, because hospitals often are units of larger organizations. Hospitals, managed care organizations, teaching institutions, and group practices must survive in a highly competitive atmosphere in which heavy emphasis is put on cost containment and increasing market share.

Put another way, to go into management today, one needs to be ready to like the challenge of hard choices and dealing with problems and issues created outside of areas under direct control. Seasoned executives are now retiring because of the change in the nature of the business. However, where such changes occur, opportunities exist for those tough enough to see the challenge as exciting, not merely dangerous.

Strategies for Entry into and Success in Management

Strategies for entry depend on formal education and the attainment of degrees. Success in management depends on being in positions with ever-increasing responsibility.

Education, Education, and Lifelong Learning

What one does first in preparing for any profession and/or complex life endeavor is usually to seek out learning opportunities related to the knowledge and skill area that one seeks to master. For medical students, this might mean acquiring some management and public health administration expertise while attending medical school, perhaps in a joint degree program. For those already past their formal education years, short courses can be helpful. Many universities already cater to physicians seeking more extensive managerial education and have programs that meet most needs.

Seek Out a Mentor

It is helpful for those in managerial roles to have someone with whom they can have candid discussions about issues, problems, and opportunities. Ideally, a physician can find someone appropriate within the institution where he or she is employed. If there is no one, it is better to seek someone from another institution or from outside the health care field but in management to assist in developing the skills.

Some organizations have deliberate policies of requiring each supervisor of an executive to take on the mentoring task. This is ensured by requiring a second mentor outside of reporting channels. A professor, a management consultant, or a former board member in a similar organization can be sought out for assistance in this role. Another physician executive who has higher-level responsibilities or works outside the institution may also be helpful. Most people are flattered when asked to play this role.

Observe, Observe, Observe

It helps to be an observer of human behavior. Most persons have ample opportunity to see what works and what does not work, merely by looking around and watching what people do. I had an opportunity to observe a very successful leader who has done outstanding work in leading committees and associations. Before I observed him, I had always wondered how he was so successful. I thought he might be too shy to make it work. However, after seeing him over an extended number of meetings, I noticed that he listened for some time, and then when he spoke up he managed to clearly identify himself with each of the major factions on issues. When it came time for closure, he clearly articulated the main concerns and related that he had, after some agonizing, come to a conclusion that he thought might yield a better result.

Watching anyone with a reputation of having mastered the art of reaching consensus is worthwhile and usually available to anyone interested in learning. If you lack access to such people, seek out someone who does and ask them to share their approaches with you. Even though I have taken a lot of graduate courses over the years, I still feel that many of my most valuable learning experiences were during personal contact with masters of the art of management.

Seek Variety in Work and Learning Experiences

There are always multiple perspectives to any management issue. The more of these perspectives you can learn, the more capable you will become in finding solutions to the problems these perspectives present. As one of my mentors has stated, how you feel about any issue depends on where you sit. In thinking about structuring the ideal apprenticeship rotation for young administrators just out of graduate school, I once recommended that a rotation, perhaps as long as three years, be established that would provide one year in a large group practice, one in hospital administration, and one with Blue Cross. Today, that apprenticeship would be one year in a vertically integrated firm, one in a large teaching hospital, and one in a managed care company. The main idea is to get the perspectives of different players in the overall scheme of financing, organizing, and delivering health care.

Take Some Risks and Volunteer

Seek out opportunities to gain new and different managerial experiences. Volunteering for committees, especially chairmanships, can bring new exposures. If exposure to managed care or quality process development, liaison roles, or other such opportunities come up, take them. If it is risky to do some of these things, in the long run it is less risky than actually taking a new position in a field with which you are unfamiliar. Reasoned approaches to risk taking, putting out the message that you are willing to take on chores and shoulder risk, and communicating that you have an interest in becoming a broader based manager are good signals to organizations looking to move people into broader roles. If you happen to be in an organization that is threatened by such behavior, take the risk, get the exposure, and move on to a more progressive organization.

Build Networks of Colleagues Traveling the Executive Path

There is probably no field that relies more on networking for colleagueship, mentoring, job opportunities, and personal growth than health administration. There are association-oriented networks, book clubs, correspondence clubs, and even research and development groups that actually serve clients even as they serve their own growth opportunities. If you do not see one readily available for you to join, create your own. I had a client once who was dying to get into one of the more exclusive clubs but simply could not. He hired me to help him and some industrial clients create a competitive club. Within six months of the development of this effort, it was canceled. He and his industrial backers were admitted to the club into which he had originally sought entry.

Literally every group you join and use to build your knowledge and skill base has within it the opportunity for building networks. Even those of us who are not big joiners can appreciate the value of such networks.

Read, Write, and Participate in Computer Network Bulletin Boards

In the early years of hospital administration, a profession for which I have taught and on which I have done research but of which I have not been a member, the rule was that the professional administrator ought to write at least two articles per year for publication. With the burgeoning numbers of graduates today, this excellent advice no longer holds. Time must be devoted to understanding the ideas that show up in business, health administration, economic development, and other, related areas of knowledge. Reading seems to be a must. Increasingly, computer networks may provide a vehicle for competing with the thoughtful letter, memorandum, and short article. My guess is that they will complement, not replace, more detailed exposition.

To these items I would add that it is also helpful to participate in other forums for idea exchange. Listening to speeches can be helpful, but working to distill and explain your own ideas in a speech can be even more of a growth experience. It produces immediate feedback.

Conclusions

On balance, today is an exciting time for executives in health care. Every organization is undergoing major change. Some forms are dying out; others are emerging. Even those succeeding today may not survive in the next few years. There is real challenge in an industry on the threshold of such change.

In some respects, the changes faced in health care mirror the changes in the air transport industry and other regulated industries that have been deregulated, such as banking. In other respects, health care is different. Medicine is the preeminent profession—independent and respected—and it is moving toward an employment situation with little opportunity for solo, private practice, or even independent small groups.

At the same time, genetics and created life forms are on the threshold of transforming medical interventions. There is not only movement to outpatient care; there is also the potential for truly new forms of care and intervention. At the other extreme, there is the possibility of an aging society overwhelming existing medical caregiving and support institutions. The time for innovation has arrived. But this is also the time of big business running medical care enterprises.

Physicians who wish to lead this revolution must become masters of management and organizational design and development. Other people can do this, but none have the potential for the same depth of insight into the underlying science and practice that are at the heart of the health care enterprise. All of these changes can be viewed as real challenges for managers and executives. On the science and medical practice front, physicians will supply major leadership. On the organization and delivery front, managers, many of them physicians, will play major roles.

Notes

1. This shift is very complex and requires more attention. For a major debate on the subjects involved, see *Health Care Management Review*, spring, summer, and fall issues, 1994, in which Richard Johnson and I, along with other authors, discuss these changes.

2. A postulate of the debate that I have had with Richard Johnson and others is that physicians can own and operate some of these for-profit businesses during a critical transition period from the entrepreneurial start-up phase until the firm is of sufficient size and scope and profitability that it then needs heavy capital infusions to grow and/or when physician owners want to convert their ownership interest into stock that has a ready market to allow them to cash out at will.

Chapter Eighteen

Provider Leadership to Promote Health

Montague Brown

Leaders who would transform the health care system and lead their communities to a better future need to look beyond the shop-worn trilogy of vertical integration, managed care, and networking. Granted, these currently are important strategies for survival for those who would maintain viability for the goals and purposes of their organizations in a changing health care economy. These are strategies that keep organizations alive. If the necessary steps have been taken to become a lean, efficient system of services covering a population base that enables a provider sufficient volume to allow the offering of a full range of services, success has been achieved. Why would anyone want to do more?

Maintaining viability in an industry whose customers are increasingly asking for better health for fewer dollars is not enough to claim a clear leadership position in the community. The demand for sick care crested in the 1980s. Though population growth and the ability of medicine to fix many problems will keep demand high, the time when unlimited resources will be thrown at insatiable demand has passed. Managed care puts heavy pressure on efficiency. Employers and governments are seeking data to assure them that real value is being delivered by the curative system. When the savings from managed care slow down, pressure will grow to find other means to reduce the nation's health bill. When the gains of efficiencies disappear, the opportunities for improvement in health status and affordability lie in domains normally outside the realm of the hospital, curative disciplines, and insurance companies. Future savings will increasingly have to come from prevention of illness and promotion of healthy lifestyles, probably using ideas from other cultures that place greater emphasis on nonclinical approaches.

The Health Repair Business Versus Prevention and Self-Healing

Health care as we know it today is in the repair business. Repair of broken bones, replacement of vital organs, and regulation of deficient systems with drugs make up the core business of what we call the health care enterprise. For what it does, it is outstanding; it is also costly, and at times wasteful. The technological basis for this form of health care is driving the debate about cost. Wars are waged against disease with magic bullets like the antimicrobial agents now on the wane as microbes mutate and overcome the overused agents.

The Chinese approach health by looking for ways to strengthen the individual's internal resistance so that harmful influences are resisted naturally by the immune system. The United States repairs, the Chinese seek to prevent. Actually, both do both, but the main strategies differ markedly. Managed care firms seem to like the idea of prevention, but they do little beyond the shots and the literature offerings on diet and exercise. Managed care firms manage the cost of the repair business, not health, healing, or prevention. They seek lower-cost treatments and only essential repair. Essentially, the U.S. "health care" system is a "sick care" system. "Health insurance" is actually "sick care insurance."

Individuals and families are responsible for their own health and for the activities and choices that promote good health. Health food stores and alternative treatments and techniques collect billions of dollars and seem to be growing, but the mainstream of American medicine turns a deaf ear to alternative strategies for pursuing improved health, as does the insurance industry and government. The idea of reducing the fat in school diets gets little assistance from mainstream health professionals, although desirable fat levels in diet are widely recognized and considered a desirable change. Such activities find no reimbursement, they offer no quick fix, and no profit—and they get no support.

The literature on the role of prevention is sparse and lacks potential solutions. Inoculations that boost the immune system's response to disease are generally acceptable. It is logical to avoid investing nonreimbursed resources in unknown areas, and because the prevailing paradigm is to treat disease, research and sponsor efforts are missing. Research dollars are not likely to be allocated to self-healing enhancements when the dominant medical and insurance paradigms exclude such inquiry.

Attempts to shed light on alternative approaches to health and self-healing are viciously attacked as voodoo science. Robert L. Park, professor of physics at the University of Maryland, writes in *The New York Times,* "Researchers in the office of alternative medicine at the National Institutes of Health espouse psychic healing and homeopathic medicine. What they [he cited others as well] all share is a profound hostility to modern science."[1] Such hostility to researching methods that seek to supplement the immune system rather than replace it with a drug is itself very shortsighted. Consider the approach being taken by Andrew Weil, author of *Spontaneous Healing:* "We are establishing a fellowship program and clinic for Integrative Medicine at the University of Arizona where we will teach alternative approaches, require Fellows to carry out research, and seek generally to integrate these less invasive and gentler approaches to the routine practice of Medicine."[2] Which is the more rational, scientific approach? Some see witches behind anything not within the currently accepted paradigm, while others see spontaneous healing (and "placebo effects" that cause healing). If these methods can be more widely used, and a new crop of medical scientists trained, the longer journey of research to sort out what works from what does not can be begun.

While Weil's approach seems logical, Arnold S. Relman, former editor of the *New England Journal of Medicine,* critiques Weil's book and dismisses it as antiscience and cultist.[3] (Judging from the number of articles in health care journals I saw just in the same week that I read Relman's review, there seems to be a concerted attempt to push back the Dark Ages, or the New Age, and to protect the existing scientific paradigm.) With all of the proposed cutbacks in Congress, those uninterested in alternative approaches to health care are still out to gut such efforts. Judging from the number of people buying Weil's book, it appears that people want more alternatives and are taking responsibility for seeking them out.

Natural healing, lifestyle, and other methods that seek to assist natural processes are rarely offered a place in the pantheon of technology, the modern hospital. Insurers have many reasons for not giving discounts for healthy lifestyles, including the pessimistic view that since 80 percent of health care expenditures are paid out in the last six months of life, healthy practices merely delay the inevitable. When asked a question about whether insurance covered the methods he used, Weil answered, "Well, we all know that what tends to be done are procedures for which reimbursement is available. The irony here is that if I recommend fifteen biofeedback sessions for hypertension, the patient will have to pay for it. If I put the patient on medication, insurance will pay for it for life!" To make more rational distinctions about what to cover, insurers need research data. To get the research, the dominant profession and research establishment must engage in the discovery process. Without that, stalemates exist. With these kinds of hurdles to overcome in considering how to do more to prevent illness and promote health, inaction or at least a strategy of benign neglect is understandable.

If one looks rationally at the incentives given health providers for prevention and health promotion, it is reasonable to conclude that no serious priority should be assigned to such activities. Given the attacks that physicians face when they try to get a hearing for alternatives, one might even argue that keeping one's job may depend on keeping away from any alternatives that challenge traditional practice. Some may ask, "Why prevent when you can make big bucks repairing failures, and repairing failed repairs pays even better."

A change in paradigm from cure to health enhancement may be long in coming. It seems unlikely to come from the mainstream of health care providers and health insurers. When things work well for any group, they are always reluctant to make changes. As with managed care, consumers and payers need to make the demands for change. Those demands are emerging.

If such thoughts are outside the mainstream, do they have any place in the array of strategies that health professionals should promote? The answer is yes. The concept of a professional connotes a primary concern for the patient, client, or customer. Ways to foster ideas and programs that promote the body's self-defense and healing systems are important. This requires reaching people in places other than our modern hospitals. It also means making a serious effort to apply good science to promising approaches. "Healing and Health" as a title for the effort would be helpful.

A second reason for promoting programs to support the body's self-defense and healing systems is to reduce the dollars spent on health. We know that people in good shape who believe in themselves and have a positive attitude about their role in their own health and recovery do better when they have episodes of illness. This translates into lower cost and leaves more dollars for profits or a lower cost for health insurance.

Prevention and health enhancement efforts are also related to the end of life, the dying and death cycle. If people learn at an early age to ward off illness and expedite recovery, they will also learn of the futility of technologically extending life for a few hours, days, or weeks. With health care financing increasingly putting the risk on health professionals, the time is already here for accepting such a philosophy of life and death. Living better and dying appropriately now has a strong financial push to become the reality.

Healthy lifestyle factors now have widespread support, but they are not reinforced in many settings. People might learn new and better ways to live if health professionals joined school boards, youth clubs, and employer groups in promoting healthy lifestyles. Health professionals could boost their image through such efforts to improve health status.

The initial leap into prevention and health promotion is easy. Everyone endorses the idea of self-responsibility for staying healthy. Having caregivers and institutions participate in community efforts is an important strategy. Since the existing health care dollar is shrinking and carries no reward for such activities, institutions need to view such work as a community and citizenship responsibility. In concert with other community leaders, institutions need to find financing for these important activities. Health professionals can influence people's decisions to try new approaches. They have the knowledge and skills needed for leadership in assisting individuals, families, organizations, and communities to become healthier.

Traditional medicine is now under fire from managed care as well as from consumers. Revenue is declining at a time when expenditures for alternative approaches, health foods, and lifestyle programs are growing. A substantial portion of this revenue should be spent with people like Weil, rather than with less well-prepared practitioners. American medicine should be providing a sounder scientific basis for alternatives.

Many alternative approaches to health care are empowering the individual. To engage in a search for ways to heal oneself and to ward off environmental insults is an empowering act. Waiting for technology and others who have the exclusive knowledge and skills to do the healing act undermines the kind of confidence needed for healing and encourages dependency. In many areas of treatment, most notably cancer, clinicians do many things to encourage patient involvement and empowerment. In these situations, the physicians are teachers and technicians. Teachers empower, and empowerment aids healing.

Now consider the other side. Those who sell services to fix things are now losing out to alternatives. Whenever heroic treatments near the end of life are avoided, providers lose additional revenue. Where drug research leads to a product that can be protected for years by patent, it is likely to attract attention. If this sounds crass and unfeeling, it is; but it also reflects an uneasy truth, that there are vast profits in using technology to prolong death.

Improving the health status of communities is not an easy goal for institutions to accept, since revenues and profits come primarily from a breakdown of health and the sale of technology for cures. It is not easy for traditional providers to package prevention as a way to lower the demand for curative services. There is little money to be made on such efforts. If insurers and managed care plans provide allowances to support such activities and lower expenditures result, they do not share the savings.

All in all, this is a rather bleak picture for prevention and alternative healing. Add to this the possibility of the promoters of prevention and alternatives being attacked as antiscience or cultist by members of a medical staff.

Finally, a major argument can be made against moving towards prevention and self-healing. The issue is opportunity cost. Having less opportunity to provide services that are no longer needed in the same amount does not favor the curative medical system. Similar to what other industries have done, one might develop "skunk works" (or experimental and developmental divisions) to protect newer ideas from traditional thinking.

On balance, the arguments for avoiding spontaneous healing are specious and short-sighted. Yes, we need evidence that this approach works. But should such alternatives be held to a higher standard than current medical practice? Today, we know from reputable scientific studies that estrogen treatment may or may not lead to higher rates of cancer, but medical practitioners are not condemned for choosing this or another approach, or for allowing the patient to decide. Physicians are not condemned for using drugs when scientific proof of their efficacy is lacking. Medicine is still part art, part science. Supporting research for alternative methods will be needed once maximum efficiencies in health care have been achieved.

Conclusions

At the hospital level, it is time to establish a program, to develop a strategy, for entering the age of integrative medicine. Few institutions are prepared to enter this arena. Given the controversy that can be anticipated, it would be best to engage in study and consensus building as a first step. Weil's program will be graduating researchers, teachers, and practitioners engaging in the kind of research needed to move this field forward. The program needs to be expanded into other regions of the country.

At the national level, self-healing needs its own institute, along with solid funding to encourage more research to validate approaches. Weil argues that such an institute should be dedicated to health and healing as well as curative medicine. He comments, "We want people who know the difference between when one works better for us than another. At this time, Americans are trying many things which have too little evidence to validate or reject the use. We need science applied to this new area, not ad hoc scare tactics to keep alternatives out of the market place of ideas."

A low fat diet, daily exercise, and other healthful activities seem to be the order of the day. When it comes to one's own health, it is wise to follow the admonition that people are first and foremost their own decision makers. Good genes are important, but need to be facilitated. Medicine can do many things, but individuals can also do many things for themselves.

It is desirable to do everything possible to keep people healthy and productive, but evidence is lacking on what works in both traditional medicine and alternatives. As more and more people seek out alternatives or supplements to traditional medicine, it will become more important for physicians to appreciate what Weil is starting at the University of Arizona. It is folly to deny the existence of scientific evidence to support alternative theories, as well as to deny the legitimacy of research into these approaches.

Notes

1. Park, Robert L. "The Danger of Voodoo Science." *The New York Times,* July 9, 1995, op-ed page.
2. This quote summarizes remarks made by Weil at a book signing and question-and-answer session held in Tucson, Arizona, July 8, 1995. Weil is a well-known author, herbalist, and faculty member of the Department of Medicine at the University of Arizona Medical School. His latest book, *Spontaneous Healing* (New York: Knopf, 1995), was number five on the best-seller list of *The New York Times Book Review* on July 9, 1995.
3. Relman, A. S. "Alternative Medicine: A Shot in the Dark." *The Wall Street Journal,* Wednesday, July 12, 1995, Leisure and Arts section.

Chapter Nineteen

New Goals for Graduate Education in Health Administration

Everett A. Johnson

As health care moves into an economic era characterized by $1 billion integrated delivery systems, the traditional curriculum of health administration needs to be rethought. The historical mission of graduate education to prepare for senior administrative positions in hospitals is rapidly becoming outdated as new graduates begin their careers in related health care organizations. Today, managed care companies, medical practice management, home health services, consulting firms, single specialty health care firms, and local, state, and federal health agencies are attracting the majority of program graduates. In addition, the large integrated health care systems are seeking graduates interested in lifelong careers in specialized management roles in their organizations.

There is an emerging need to restructure health administration curriculums to meet the functionally specialized administrative staffing needs of the large health care systems and the needs of health care related entities. The view that one specific health administration curriculum is adequate to prepare all graduates is not responsive to the needs of the field. There is now an opportunity to bring other university resources to bear on specific educational tracks to prepare students for more specialized administrative careers in health care. As integrated systems mature and stabilize their internal operations, they will need, as major components of their organizations, people who have chosen long-term careers as senior managers.

The expansion of health care systems into organizations that combine physician services with several levels of patient care facilities, resulting in multiple parent-subsidiary levels that are geographically dispersed, will require senior managers who understand the unique administrative requirements of health care and who have in-depth knowledge and specialized organizational skills for managing finance, marketing, information systems, insurance, human resources, operations, or managed care. Several senior executives will need to be cross-trained in both health administration and a business specialty area. Typically, these positions will be at the vice presidential level and will involve directing the major support services of marketing, managed care, information systems, finance, human resources, operations management, and real estate operations. When a health system needs to fill one of these senior positions, it will face a dilemma: it can either hire a person with specialized knowledge and help that person to understand the peculiarities of health care administration, or it can select an existing staff person and provide training in the specialized area. Either choice is less than desirable, and future competency is often problematic.

These changes that require different technical skills for senior managers provide an opportunity for health administration programs to develop curriculums that prepare graduates for lifetime careers in specialized senior administrative positions. Future graduates will likely have a different career path than the traditional pattern of administrative assistant to vice president of a major hospital division to chief executive officer, with eventual relocation to a larger hospital. A likely career path in a large health care system will begin in a specialized area of health administration such as a managed care company or group practice management, followed by progressive moves to larger organizations; or it will begin in a specialty administrative position, with subsequent moves to larger systems.

Preparing Future Graduates

To prepare program graduates for their new roles, curriculums must stay abreast of changes in the delivery of medical care. Recognition of new career goals is of growing importance as integrated systems expand and need senior executives with nontraditional preparation for the emerging specialized responsibilities. Traditionally, graduate programs have prepared students for administrative positions that required a generalist's knowledge. As hospitals consolidate, traditional administrative positions are disappearing and specialized administrative positions are increasing. It is clear that the majority of future graduates will have career opportunities in specialty areas.

To continue only the present curriculum in the belief that students can adjust to managing specialized areas of operation is to fail to prepare students appropriately for their future careers. The primary educational goal of a program should be preparation of students for major responsibilities in organizations that deliver medical care. When new needs arise in the field, health administration programs have an educational responsibility to respond.

In the future, graduate health administration programs should provide multiple curriculum tracks in preparation for technical administrative responsibilities in health care systems. By coupling various business concentrations with a common core of health administration knowledge, the student's time in the program can be more productive, and the expertise they develop will be more focused. At the same time, the traditional curriculum, which prepares generalists, should be available for students choosing a path leading to a chief executive position.

When a program offers students a choice in selecting a curriculum, the faculty has a responsibility to advise them about the career consequences of their choice. Older entering students, in their late twenties or thirties, who have significant work experience, typically have clear career objectives in mind, while younger students, who are one or two years past their undergraduate experience, will require counseling to establish specific career goals, such as in the following two examples:

- A twenty-three-year old fascinated with the potential for computer information applications, whose father is a physician and whose mother is a nurse, has decided that being a physician will not be a personal goal. However, he still desires a career in health care and has worked since graduation for a health information system company. Clearly, this student is a candidate for the master of science in health administration (MSHA) degree with a concentration in information systems.

- A thirty-one-year-old has a bachelor of business administration degree and has worked as the office manager of a hospital for the last eight years. The current mergers of hospitals have created an opportunity for him to be selected for a position in the finance officer's staff in the parent hospital organization. The MSHA degree with a finance concentration would be the obvious suggestion.

The primary responsibility of a program's faculty is to assist students in getting started in whatever career they choose. A secondary but important role is to impress students with the need to continue their learning throughout their working life by reading the literature of the field. A faculty must prepare graduates for both tomorrow and twenty years from now. Unless students acquire self-education habits during their campus years, within five years they will be out-of-date in a milieu that is rapidly changing and whose future is unknown.

The Responsibilities of Graduate Programs

Graduate programs will be the major source of future leaders in health administration. As the number of hospitals has decreased in the past decade, the traditional program goal of preparing students to be chief operating officers and chief executive officers has likewise been shrinking. As a result, recent graduates are beginning their work experience as department directors or in assistant positions in specialized areas of hospital or health system operations.

Graduate programs need to recognize that ad hoc adjustments of new graduates to specialized managerial responsibilities are a less-than-ideal way to embark on an administrative career. A more desirable way is to use university resources to provide curriculum tracks that more adequately prepare students for these evolving positions. Specialized curriculum tracks that couple the core curriculum of health administration with a functional business specialty area and lead to an MSHA degree with a designated specialty would meet the emerging needs of the field. A curriculum with functional specialty choices is appealing to graduate students and their future employers because it develops greater depth of knowledge and skills in the specialty areas. These educational options should be attractive to potential applicants because the length of time in graduate school, the focused effort, and the costs would be less than for a traditional health administration degree aimed at preparation of generalists.

Because the curriculum to prepare students for a generalist position has been expanded in the past decade to a three-year curriculum awarding both a master of business administration (MBA) degree and a master of health administration (MHA) degree, a more focused curriculum is desirable for a much larger group of applicants than can be accomplished in two years.

Availability of specialized health administration tracks would enable the expanding integrated health care systems to staff positions for which it is currently difficult to recruit qualified applicants. Over time, these health care systems may decide to provide specialized administrative residencies as a low-cost way of assessing the skill levels of new graduates, in order to meet their own system needs.

Elements of Specialized Curriculum Tracks

To provide concentrated curriculum tracks for MSHA degrees, a graduate program must either be a unit within a college of business administration or have access to departments in business schools with adequate faculty to offer a sufficient number of courses in the specialty area. To provide several specialty tracks requires enough faculty members to have enough courses to justify each functional specialty. It is likely that only colleges of business administration of substantial size will sponsor MSHA degrees with specialty concentrations.

Health administration program graduates with an MSHA degree and a field of concentration will have much better insight into how to operate the major services of health care organizations in an integrated fashion in order to provide more efficient support. As integrated health care systems expand in size and number of delivery sites, they will need to decentralize the decision-making structure, thus providing greater authority for senior executive positions in order to provide cost-effective patient care services. In this type of operating environment, technical skill and an understanding of health administration will be essential. The core courses for the health administration curriculum can be more limited for the specialized tracks than for the generalist track that leads to MBA and MHA degrees.

The goal of the core health administration curriculum is to create a framework for understanding the interrelationship of organizational goals and support services goals. With an understanding of the larger health care issues and the restraints affecting medical care delivery, many present-day managers can transform their traditional parochial viewpoint into a cooperative attitude that comes from a broader grasp of the key issues.

To prepare students for graduate work in either business or health administration requires some foundation courses prior to matriculation. Students will need to know how to use algebra and statistics and they will need a basic familiarity with accounting, in addition to understanding the concepts of microeconomics and the fundamentals of organization and administrative theory. Students in the specialized health administration tracks can be more selective than for the generalist track. Specialty health administration students will need an understanding of the economics of health care and the unique legal doctrines of medical care. In order to integrate the practice of their specialty area with the other parts of the health care system, they will need to know how to integrate and cooperate with other parts of a delivery system.

The curriculum for each specialized area is a set of related courses that provide students with a basic set of skills that are typical of other masters students in each of these fields. At graduation a student should be sufficiently skilled to perform satisfactorily at the associate level in a major support service operation for a large integrated system.

A set of related courses for a specialty area would usually be directed and staffed by separate departments within a college of business administration. The number of departmental courses to be included and identified as a major or concentration area for the MSHA degree would vary by department specialty, and also according to the degree awarding policies of the college. Because they are blended with health administration courses, the total number of specialty courses would likely exceed the requirement for a master of science in the specialty field.

There are within each department specific courses that provide a basic set of skills and knowledge to adequately prepare students for positions in specialized support services. These graduates would not have sophisticated technical skills; rather, they would have a detailed understanding of the methodology and concepts of the specialty and how they are applied. The first position for graduates would likely be a job as an assistant in a regional health care organization or as an associate director in a smaller operation.

For each specialty area there are specific departmental courses that teach the skills and knowledge needed in health care organizations:

Managed Care. The key concepts and strategies of managed care are taught by risk management and insurance departments. Courses deal with risk analysis and control, managed competition, health insurer operations, and employee benefit planning. The concepts of managed care are fundamentally insurance methodologies applied to health care cost control. When this information is coupled with the material taught in health administration courses, a student is provided with the knowledge base for understanding the integration of risk and insurance practice to direct managed care operations. It would also be useful for students to enroll in one or two actuarial courses to gain a more detailed grasp of underwriting strategies.

Marketing. The curriculum to prepare for managing a marketing operation would include how to do market research, buyer behavior, communications, promotion, and strategic market planning. The abilities to design a marketing strategy, to gather and interpret results, to affect individual and family decision making, and to market to health care consumers are the goals of a marketing curriculum. Customer orientation and pricing considerations will become increasingly important as health care systems compete for patients.

Information Systems. An executive with an understanding of the structure and operation of a health care system is needed to apply information system concepts to developing a useful database, designing and integrating a network, and determining its specifications. A graduate would need to be prepared to analyze and design information systems; to develop communications for both local and wide-area networks; to integrate hardware, software, and management services; and to conduct training programs.

Finance. As large health care systems evolve, a chief financial officer will need expertise in corporation financing, managerial accounting and control, corporate capital structures, financial management of operations, and health care financing. As investor-owned systems are created from nonprofit organizations, there will be issues about dividend policies, capital structure strategies, and market valuation of stock prices. A health administration background will be needed to accommodate the key role of physicians in controlling medical care through appropriate financial mechanisms in the organization.

Human Resources. The responsibility for managing the human resources of large, multilocation staffs and assuring compliance with certification and licensing requirements, position content analysis, and appraising performance will require a knowledge of both the unique requirements for health care personnel and legal restraints. An understanding of organizational behavior, industrial relations, employee benefit planning, staff training, and wage and salary administration will become increasingly complex.

Real Estate Management. As a health system expands its facilities throughout its service area, whether on an owned or leased basis, it will require a senior executive who can fit the organization's strategy to its real estate needs. A knowledge of the financing of real estate, planning and developing projects, and how to deal with the legal and regulatory environment when acquiring property will be essential as a system's service demands shift over time.

Operations Management. The integration of multiple operations will require improved decision methodologies for resource allocation and scheduling. These methodologies will be based on computer simulation models to achieve improvements in both quality and productivity. Knowledge of both health administration and business forecasting methods will be required.

Each of these areas of management specialization will require a level of expertise that is not possible to achieve in a curriculum that prepares generalists in health administration. Traditional health administration in the future will experience a gradual reduction in job opportunities for their graduates as the number of generalist positions in hospitals declines. However, there will also be an increase in the number of positions established to manage physician group practices, which will need the skills of traditional course graduates.

Conclusions

In the future, the source of chief executive officers for the large, regional health care delivery systems will not be limited to any particular type of educational track in health administration. It is likely that no particular pattern will be followed; rather, similarly to the pattern of commercial business, selections will be made to fit the current needs of the firm. When a business is weak in its marketing functions or has serious financing problems, it typically selects a new chief executive whose strength is in the area of the company's greatest need.

This same pattern will emerge in health care. Where there are clinical problems, a physician will be selected; for managed care difficulties, an experienced managed care executive will be chosen. The path to the golden ring will be based on previous experience and outstanding performance. Graduate programs should not be concerned with preparing students for their long-term career goals. Instead, to benefit current and emerging executive needs in health care, graduate programs should establish goals that will meet the needs of the field in the immediate future.

Part Five

Conclusion

Chapter Twenty

Now to the Real Change

Montague Brown

The tooth fairy is loose again. To Mr. and Ms. America, managed care via capitation will mean rationing of access. No longer will providers speak of high quality. They will speak of acceptable quality, affordability, and essential care—not care on demand. We are indeed well into this economic era. We have gone far, with farther yet to go. This book has recounted how we moved here. Much of what is recounted is easy to agree with. Much more, however, needs to be explored if we are to fully grasp the meaning of this shift.

From Alms to Technology

The movement of medical services and hospitals has been from sick houses for the poor operated by the wealthy to technological marvels whose services are demanded by everyone and sold in the marketplace by national firms whose stock is traded daily on Wall Street. Wall Street is a rock-solid American institution whose goal is the old fashioned profits expected by every successful business. As we move down the road to rationing health care, managed care firms funded by Wall Street equity and debt will prosper. They will meet the need for business and government to offer choice while at the same time constraining resource use. Voluntary hospitals

Note: This chapter has been adapted from Brown, M. "The Economic Era: Now to the Real Change." *Health Care Management Review,* 1994, *19*(4), 73–81. Copyright © 1994, Aspen Publishers, Inc. Used with permission.

and their trustees will be ill-equipped to ration care, given their bedrock value of succoring the poor while lavishing compassionate, high-tech care on all patients, all the while being reimbursed, whatever the cost. Paradigms may shift but institutions rarely adapt. More often than not they are replaced. Not many buggy companies became automobile firms. Railroad firms rarely see themselves as being in the air freight or over-the-road transportation business. Old concepts are, in reality, straitjackets.

In the course of the transition of hospitals from alms houses to technological marvels, and now into the economic era, health insurance has shifted from a pass-through insurance mechanism to a system in which utilization is aggressively managed and controlled and competitively priced, in a manner that determines which providers get to provide services to which patients. Further, the controls also determine when, where, and how patients may get services, if and when they are to be provided. In very little time, we have moved light years away from patients choosing whichever doctor and hospital they desire whenever they decide they need one. For America, it may be rationing time.

Charity care was replaced by cost shifting. The alms house was all charity. But as the poor and the paying began to go to the same hospital, cost shifting became the major mode of financing charity care. Cost shifting continues today, as governments shift costs to employers, and large employers in turn shift costs to small employers, who in turn shift costs to individual buyers. It is little wonder that there is an insurance and financing crisis. Managed care will leave this cost shifting in place. Economic muscle counts, and the government has the biggest clout. Maybe we would all be better off enrolling in either Medicare or the Federal Employees Health Benefit Plan. The woes of the postal system notwithstanding, government health care might be preferable. If we are going to have managed care either way, why not use the profits to reduce the national debt rather than have it go to Wall Street?

Richard Johnson pointed to 1990 as the time when capital needs and balanced budgets became driving forces in hospitals. I would place that date somewhere in the late 1960s and mid 1970s, when Medicare and Medicaid "promised" to pay for the care of all or most of the needy. Remember that during those early days, Congress acted as though health care was a right, even though they never got around to funding it as such. Once debt financing was well-established, in the 1970s, voluntary hospitals were captive to the financial ratio analysis of bond rating agencies. If hospitals wanted access to debt capital operating and financial ratios, they had to follow a business pattern. For the boards of directors of many successful hospitals, bond ratings are important indicators of success.

Some people attribute the advent of the economic era of hospitals to the development of the investor-owned chain. While this was a factor, the debt financing of not-for-profit hospitals did much to ensure this shift. Ironically, many of the innovations in financing of not-for-profit hospitals are attributable to the financial ingenuity of investor-owned chains.

During the 1980s, a business or economic orientation became entrenched at hospitals, and in the mid 1990s few if any hospitals are left in which the driving force is the view that community good and charity are primary. This does not mean that no one talks about such concepts anymore, but it does mean that talk is, after all, merely talk. Even the rare trustee who may vote against cost cutting and rationing of services knows that to lose contracts only results in fewer patients for a hospital in a competitive environment.

The economic era will fundamentally change medical practice in this country. Physician practice styles, their businesses, and their autonomy are under siege. Integration of physicians with other providers poses both threats and opportunities. Many hospitals and health care systems are establishing partnerships utilizing physician-hospital organizations (PHOs), MSOs, and/or wholly owned practice groups. Insurers are seeking to build a controlled primary care base while limiting contracts with hospitals and specialists. Hospital-based integrated systems usually suffer from including too many specialists. At the same time, insurers may have a too-restricted panel of specialists.

Physicians seem to be at risk from both hospitals and insurers. Physicians who join group practices with a primary care base of 50 percent or more, and who expand regionally to serve contiguous markets, have tremendous leverage potential. One group in California bought a small hospital, expanded covered lives to more than one hundred thousand, and then contracted for specialty services from a university hospital on a fixed rate for ten beds plus services. This amounted to only one hundred beds for a population of one million. Over a ten-year period, The Lovelace Clinic doubled its number of covered lives and physicians while keeping bed capacity at the same level. Lovelace is now owned by an insurance carrier that evolved from a combined group practice and not-for-profit hospital. Both participants grew as they obtained access to capital markets. Physicians and hospitals throughout the country are now duplicating this effort. Many physician owners need equity capital to convert fixed assets to liquid assets. Equity markets provide this liquidity to physicians. Many locally owned not-for-profit organizations cannot provide physicians with the kind of return on assets that can be commanded in a public equity market.

Financial Characteristics of the Economic Era

There is no doubt that the era under way is associated with consolidation and competition. Other indicators of the era are the growing number of investor-owned and tax-paying entities, as well as economic partnerships among physicians and various organizations that own and operate physician practices, albeit under a variety of guises. In the economic era, profit means more than just the capital necessary to grow, replace, and innovate; profit is increasingly a personal motivator that results in individual riches. This is a far different motivator than existed in the benevolent years of health care and, subsequently, during the technological era.

The desire of purchasers of insurance and benefits (businesses, governments, and to a lesser extent, individuals) is to achieve better value for their premium dollars. The buyers are not the patients; government is not the patient. They are the entities that want relief. They want physician fees slashed, hospital costs capped, and everything cost managed. They are willing to pay managed care firms a good price if they will ratchet down the use of medical care resources. They demand cost containment. Managed care is the seeming salvation of the private sector; ration access, it says. The economic era is about pleasing business and government buyers. Managed care firms view business and government as customers, as do provider groups. Patients' desires must be considered, but this does not mean that care, service, and choice will be available on demand.

There are other proximate causes of the cost problem. Community hospitals compete by utilizing the latest and best that technology can offer. Physicians also thrive on this concept in the fee-for-service arrangement. Federal policy initially contributed to this situation when fee-for-service was adopted for Medicare and Medicaid. Medicare began with cost-plus reimbursement. Later, it merely paid cost. And now, for many providers Medicare pays below cost, but even with this change, Medicare may still be a profit center.

In order to keep up technologically, hospitals turned to the bond markets in a major way. With financial results practically guaranteed through cost reimbursement, the bond markets eagerly responded with debt offerings, since a good time and great profits were to be had by all. Equity markets responded to for-profit hospital chains, managed care firms, and physician management companies. Equity and market debt now promise ways to bring physicians into more ownership positions, even as the field of practice is increasingly becoming salaried under managed care firms, which often are both owned and operated by insurance firms.

As a result of investments in hospitals and other health care entities, a health care infrastructure exists that is the envy of the marketplace. The health care system could service much of the world with the capacity it has in place today. This excess capacity does, however, portend the next round of change, which will complete the cycle into the economic era: excess capacity will make price competition among hospitals and specialty physicians inevitable.

Overcapacity provides the basis for buyer-driven price competition. Simply put, when a commodity is in surplus, buyers extract price concessions. We now have a buyer's market and buyers are soliciting bids. Price competition makes it possible for insurers and managed care firms to profit initially from price discounting without changing the manner in which care is actually delivered. After extracting initial gains from price discounting, more selective contracting and the increasing use of rationing devices to control patient use of resources will be required. Thus, the new era is dawning.

All of the marketplace tools are being rolled into place to move health care into a much more competitive mode. Managed care firms and aggressive corporate buyers are driving the early stages. As hospitals and physicians realize their fate, they will move to eliminate the intermediaries and sell their own services. Hospitals and physicians will be in two camps: in one camp they will benefit from fee-for-service, and in the other they will benefit from rationing access to services. One camp will pay for resource use, the other will pay for nonuse of resources, a tough balancing act.

Insurers and providers are all seeking to position themselves to take advantage of this market shift. There is a difference between (1) the sellers, who own and operate the risk taking operation, the providers, and the marketing infrastructure, and (2) those hospitals and physicians who are merely contractors to managed care organizations, seeking to manage entire networks through contracts only.

Managed care firms benefit from price discounting by those entities that own hard assets. Hospitals, for example, face the prospect of an ever-increasing downward price spiral. Worse yet, the managed care firm may give bonuses and preferred prices to primary care physicians whose practice inclination is to minimize the use of hospital and specialty resources; thus, the hospital will be put in a unique bind, because its former colleagues will become rationing agents for its services. Such practices are especially hard on specialists and hospitals in the transition to the economic era.

Patient Responsibility

In the managed care era, patients have less responsibility than in previous eras. The capitation method places a heavy responsibility on providers to effectively ration care to patients. However, a variety of financial incentives also confront users of managed care. Many health maintenance organizations (HMOs) have disincentives to utilize services, such as co-payments and deductibles, in addition to their other methods of rationing services; and for those systems that allow patients to go outside the plan (point-of-service options), there may be a co-payment of 50 percent or even higher.

Managed care patients face great behavioral modification exercises. Since patients often present themselves to physicians with self-correcting problems, the primary contact for many may be with nonphysicians. Patients learn early on that a registered

nurse or licensed practical nurse may be the first person to inter-
cede in an episode of illness. This meeting may be followed by
meetings with a nurse practitioner or physician's assistant. These
encounters may consist of the practitioner or assistant offering sym-
pathy, followed by the patient being prescribed medication and
then scheduling a visit with the physician for two to three weeks
later. Why so long? After two weeks, a self-correcting problem will
have been resolved and no visit will be necessary. This system works
when the problem actually is self-correcting; but when it is not, the
system is problematic. This type of access rationing lowers resource
use and makes it possible for the HMOs to staff for serious clinical
needs and not for symptomatic needs.

Over time, patients learn how to "game" this type of system and
move up in the queue, but this puts a new level of burden of proof
on patients. Being on the wrong end of the rationing decision is
time consuming and may adversely affect clinical outcomes.

In some cases, the insured often pays a percentage of billed
charges while the insurer or managed care plan pays a portion as a
percentage of negotiated discounts. After deducting the full
amount of the co-payment, some insured patients, through their
co-payments, may actually pay 60 to 100 percent of what the
providers receive for their services.

Capitation

Under capitation, physicians may find ways to generate sufficient
profits by not providing services or by providing them through
physician extenders (that is, nurse practitioners or physician's assistants). This practice advances the long-held belief that capitation
provides incentives for withholding care rather than providing
care. If physicians' behavior were analyzed, the results would suggest that they might work less under capitation, that under capitation they might take more leisure time and work fewer hours since
no additional fees would be generated by working longer hours.
Conversely, any organization that has workers whose workloads are
reduced by technology (such as managed care methodologies) will
take steps to reduce the number of people in that work force.
Fewer encounters per physician ultimately means that fewer physicians will be needed.

Many of the managed care plans capitate the primary care physicians' fees and require that access to specialists, whose fees may or may not be capitated, be regulated. If specialists' fees are capitated, they are the lucky ones. Fewer specialists are needed. The idea that physicians will be paid the same amount for less and less work is simply too good to be true.

There seems to be universal acceptance by the public that there is a surplus of specialists but a shortage of primary care physicians. Knowing that the driver of managed care is profit and that the goal of purchasers is to reduce costs, managed care firms have to lower their premium charges to buyers, which forces the managed care firms to cut their costs further in order to make profits. The logical end of this downward pressure is that physicians and hospitals will be pushed for better productivity while being denied the opportunity to perform more and more procedures.

Why would physicians work long hours under capitation when it offers fewer incentives than fee-for-service for like effort? One major reason is that managed care firms own the right to assign patients to physicians. If physicians can find a sufficient volume of patients only through managed care firms, they will receive only limited income from private practice and fee-for-service.

Just as a managed care firm adjusts downward its reimbursement to hospitals, so too will it adjust upward the number of physicians on its physician panel. The principle behind capitation is to shift the incentive from resource use on demand to utilization based on health status of patients. However, in the present stage of managed care, price competition has been the real driver, rather than an attempt to manage health status. The theory of capitation calls for increasing the resources for prevention and wellness. This does not happen in the short-term. Such efforts takes years to pay off. Cutting costs through prevention may be an elusive dream. For managed care firms to invest in the long-term in order to improve the health status of entire populations, they may have to use a percentage of the fees they typically pay out to providers. To do so may require a pooling of money among managed care plans.

To date, capitation and managed care have focused on providing less-costly and more efficiently delivered and deliberately rationed access to reasonably good-quality medical services. Aside from the group and staff model of capitated arrangements, this approach has yet to be fully tested. In prepaid group practices, the concept of capitation and managed care can and does work well.

When used properly, capitation results in a shift of emphasis from early and extensive use of all types of physicians to the rationed use of specialists. The resulting difference in cost is huge. Lowered costs of care can result in large profits for self-insured employers, as well as for managed care firms that shift the capitation risks to the providers.

The potential of profits from risk shifting has led to a major race for control over the premium dollar. Opportunities for those who are in a position to profit from replacing fee-for-service by capitation is enormous. In a market glutted with providers, managed care plans can ratchet down costs and usage. The result is windfall profits, except in those states that regulate or control profits.

The PHO movement enables hospitals and physicians to realign ownership of revenue. Profits stream into a joint venture, which may enable physicians to be better compensated. Hospitals provide the majority of assets to a joint venture, but this does not necessarily mean that they will end up with majority control of the health care system.

Physicians typically constitute 20 percent or less of the hospital governing board, but in PHOs they may constitute 50 percent. Jointly owned and operated PHOs negotiate prices with buyers and managed care firms. Having an intimate knowledge of the factors involved should permit physicians to notch up their prices while shifting hospital prices down a notch. This shifting can occur because physicians are the ultimate decision makers on how much of a hospital's resources go into patient care. Where hospital fees are capitated, physicians determine nearly all hospital costs by their individual utilization patterns. Many hospitals are buying primary care practices so that they can pressure specialists in the use of hospital resources.

Under managed care, the ownership of assets becomes less important than control of the revenue streams. If the power to strike a deal is shared by a hospital and physicians, then the base of power for revenue allocation shifts. PHOs shift power away from hospital governing boards to physicians and hospital executives because the PHO is where all of the important decisions are made. This really moves governance into a professionally dominated (managers and physicians) arena. Under such circumstances, voluntary boards are at risk of becoming appendages presiding over the husk of an outmoded business enterprise.

In a health care market with surplus assets, the power to dictate is exercised by those with premium revenues but no assets to protect. Buyers dominate and large profits are realized by forcing asset owners to grant substantial price discounts. As market competition leads to hospital failures and greater consolidation among hospitals, the balance between buyers and sellers will continue to shift. Some providers will acquire an insurance function while some insurers will acquire provider functions. This will likely lead to mergers and consolidations between insurer managed care firms and major provider organizations. Perhaps five years from now the nation will have fully vertically integrated firms serving all major markets. Whether this development will lead to oligopoly pricing and control or more competition remains to be seen. In the short run, hospitals, insurers, and multispecialty groups will compete aggressively to buy up the primary care capacity in order to gain power and leverage with the other players.

The power in physician-driven organizations may eventually be shifted to publicly owned corporations, since very few if any physician groups will have amassed sufficient capital reserves to fund a move to control managed care (the large not-for-profit Mayo Clinic and a few others are exceptions). If physicians move aggressively and early into ownership roles, the corporations they establish will ultimately become publicly owned, in order to take advantage of equity financing sources.

Physician-driven entities will earn their revenues from physicians' practices and by lowering the portion of premiums allocated to hospitals. By progressively squeezing hospitals, physician groups will eventually acquire one or more hospitals. This ownership will permit maximized control over both practice revenues and profits. To accomplish this, physician entities will ultimately require outside capital that will most likely come from the deep pockets of insurers or shareholders. Those hospital systems that are able to provide physicians with an ownership interest will attract physicians by selling equity shares for recapturing the profits from their investment. Once the initial round of physician movement into salaried positions occurs, new physicians just coming into the medical field will be salaried. By then, patients will be "owned" by managed care organizations and will only be available to physicians who join the organization's networks. Future generations of physicians will only be employed by established plans because they will be unable to establish a practice outside of managed care controls.

Additional Issues to Explore

Capitation will not solve all of the major problems in health care. There are social, environmental, and economic problems that will be outside the purview of health care. Problems of poverty, drug addiction, homelessness, and other cultural matters lie beyond the rationing of access to health care services. Children having children exacerbates the health system's problems. Mothers who fail to obtain prenatal care often have troubled pregnancies; children are born prematurely, and often receive little stimulation and nurturing during their early years. The result is that a normal productive life fails to take place. Enrolling a one-parent family in an HMO does little to change this outcome. Merely controlling the cost through rationing of access may even make matters worse.

Education and research are particularly at risk in a cost-driven competitive system that does not readily support them. Cross-subsidies (sources that helped subsidize these important activities) are lacking that were available from fee-for-service payments when patients were free to choose academic physicians. In addition, the location of Veterans Administration hospitals adjacent to academic centers added both support and referrals.

Long-term disabilities (such as Alzheimer's disease) require long-term care, home care, and respite care. Such services fall outside the usual HMO contract. While many elderly and disabled persons remain at home and not in long-term care facilities, more attention and financial support are needed to encourage physical fitness in order to prevent even greater use of long-term care.

Lifestyle changes do not lend themselves to year-to-year payoffs in the performance measures that most HMOs can undertake. There are interventions that could be helpful. The Department of Agriculture recently announced a plan to change the fat content requirements for school lunches, a move aimed at preventing disabilities. Another long-term program would be a national physical fitness program. These types of policies are favorable to controlling health care costs, but they lie outside the normal scope of an HMO. Support from government for these activities would require the establishment of public policy departments. The costs of prevention and lifestyle changes do not belong in the budgets of the hospitals and specialists who contract with HMOs because the role of hospitals and specialists is to "fix illness." Those in health care who profit from prevention activities are the managed care plans that support wellness activities that ultimately reduce the costs of care. Capitation drives these programs out of hospital budgets, but it adds to the profit margins of managed care plans.

These issues are social problems and should not be loaded onto the providers of the health care delivery system. Even though health care institutions by law must provide services when people present themselves at emergency rooms for acute care, the wellness aspect should be costs borne by those organizations that benefit by their support. If wellness is not supported by governmental and managed care plans, the large public hospitals and teaching hospitals will continue to bear the brunt of providing services.

Public health advocates often fault the medical care system, including hospitals, for not being sufficiently interested in the issues outlined here. Prevention remains a token program for most health care organizations. Health maintenance organizations might be expected to take a more visible role. But will they? Will they do it only for their defined populations? Will investor-owned HMOs use corporate profits for long-term, problematic, or questionable outcomes?

Over the past few years, some hospitals have taken on advocacy and involvement in community development activities. In an intensely competitive environment, these hospitals will be squeezed by cost-driven contracts. Their only option will be to cut programs in order to survive. These issues will be part of the price paid for driving the health care system into free-market price competition.

Some hospital advocates who are taking on responsibility for community development may point to Kaiser Permanente or Henry Ford Hospital as examples to be copied. However, neither of these two organizations are models for most hospitals, for two important reasons. First, each was well-capitalized at the outset by a wealthy industrialist—Henry Kaiser and Henry Ford, respectively.

In addition, both organizations are integrated as single economic entities, which makes them profoundly different from those integrated systems that are held together by contracts. When systems are integrated by contracts—one for the hospitals, one for primary care physicians, and one for specialists—only the managed care plan stands to benefit. If a contract hospital receives a capitated rate that turns out at the end of the fiscal year to have resulted in a substantial profit because the hospital has not been used by managed care patients, it is a sure bet that the capitation rate will be reduced in the following year by the managed care plan. It may be suggested that moving from nonprofit to for-profit status will replace community service with greed and will change a profession to a commodity-type business. We fail to see this dark side. Most physicians care a great deal about their patients and regard the financial aspects as a secondary concern, yet clearly they are for-profit. With increasing frequency, hospital administrators move back and forth between for-profit and nonprofit hospitals without losing their sense of values. On any number of occasions, nonprofit hospital administrators have been heard to respond to the question, "How's your hospital doing?" with the statement, "Just great; last year we made X millions of dollars on the bottom line." It seems to us that blurs the distinction between for-profit and nonprofit.

Can hospitals avoid being pushed out of the community service role? Will trustees of nonprofit hospitals rise to the occasion and remain true to their community concerns, or will the competitive environment be so pervasive and revenues so restricted that hospitals will forego this role as they struggle for financial survival?

Conclusions

Ultimately, this book must be judged by the readers and the marketplace. The questions that readers will need to ask include the following:

- Is this book on target? Can the eventual demise of the solo public and community not-for-profit hospital be reasonably predicted? If hospital systems cannot or will not aggressively transform themselves into health care systems with a tightly managed care arm, will they survive?

- If managed care becomes fully integrated with physicians and capitated reimbursement becomes the norm, is it possible to predict the gradual assumption by physicians of the top executive functions in such systems? Does this mean that hospitals will increasingly come under the overall management and/or direction of physicians because of clinically driven protocols? The theory for this postulate predicts that when a profession is overtaken by bureaucracy, the professionals will seek to control the bureaucracy and thus their own destiny. Physician demand for equality in governance is an example.
- Will the need for market capital for physicians' practices, managed care entities, and investor-owned hospitals result in the eventual dominance of for-profit enterprises in health care? A number of teaching hospitals are now contemplating the conversion of their hospitals into for-profit entities, similar to what the Lovelace Clinic did ten years ago.
- If more and more of health care is for-profit, will this result in a loss of tax-exempt status for many hospitals? If governments look favorably on those who pay taxes, will hospitals with tax-exempt status receive much more careful scrutiny?
- If health reform moves toward universal coverage, will the not-for-profits have even less of an argument for a preferred status?
- Since physicians can legally participate in equity holdings, will they not pressure nonprofit hospitals to spin off the hospital business to allow them an ownership interest? Consulting firms are already offering to implement models that spin off the hospital, convert the assets to for-profit status, and sell the physicians equity interests in the newly created entity.
- How far up the chain, from community hospital to teaching hospital to academic medical center, is this change likely to go? Will large physician groups like Scripps, Mayo Clinic, and Cleveland Clinic shift from not-for-profit to for-profit in order to maintain market share and to share in the rewards that come from tightly controlled managed care?

The major rewards for tightly controlled managed care occur in the early years. If managed care plans have windfall profits, buyers will continue to exert more and more downward pressure.

Managed care plans are undoubtedly aware of this possibility. When it happens, managed care plans will seek to cut their own costs further. The degree to which this will occur will depend on the amount of competition remaining in the marketplace.

The health care system is now in the throes of being shifted into a managed care mode. Medicaid and Medicare may also be pushed into the same risk pools in order to satisfy buyers. Some purchasers of care do seek value through cost benefit, but for most buyers the goal is lower prices. Increasing co-payments and deductibles and rationing access through capitation are viewed as the way of avoiding unnecessary use of resources. Though unspoken, this approach relies on the self-correcting nature of illness and the willingness of people to live with discomfort.

The emerging institutions and organizations may well be required to fit the business mentality of Wall Street. Like the buggy manufacturer who was replaced by the automobile firm, community institutions will likely yield to tough-minded business management. Some nonprofit organizations will transform themselves, but many are likely to fail.

This transformation is going on now. How will the American people respond to these changes? My coauthors and I suspect that they will be accepted in theory but ultimately resented in practice. Rather than wait to find out who will be the winners and the losers, now is the time to place bets, pick sides, and do something about your favorite policy direction. Which way will it all go?

In the final analysis, we hope that community mission will survive. If it does not, the American public will be the loser.

Index

A

Academic teaching hospital: physicians in management of, 239; trends for, 36

Accountability, for providers and insurers, 146

Accreditation, and ethics, 96, 102, 140, 146–147

Affiliations: aspects of, 21–39; attractiveness of, 231–232; background on, 21–23; breaking up, 80; and competition, 189–190; conclusions on, 37–38; and contracts, 200; future for, 34–37; and governance, 164–166, 168–169, 176–177; history of, 23–27; of hospitals, 27–29, 164–166, 168–169; and ideas, 22; and managed care, 29–34; and partner selection, 111–112; reasons for, 107; trends for, 78–80, 89

American College of Surgeons, 140

American Health Association (AHA), 30, 39

American Health Systems, 25, 27

American Hospital Association, 45n, 46, 83n, 91

American Medical Association, 20

Anders, G., 116, 130

Antitrust laws, and hospitals, 26, 36, 90

Arizona, University of, Integrative Medicine at, 252, 257

Autonomy: individual, 210–211; local, 209–210

B

BJC, as regional system, 37

Blue Cross and Blue Shield: and catastrophic coverage, 62, 64; commercialization of, 197–198; and managed care, 124; and minimum benefits, 66; and physicians as managers, 239; trends for, 35, 77, 118

Board: as collective authority, 159–161; composition of, 167; consolidated, 213–214; executive committee of, 160; for integrated systems, 211–215; measuring, 162–163; nominating and evaluating committee of, 162–163; of nonprofit hospitals, 80; responsibility of, 161, 174, 175, 176, 183; role of, 156–157, 187–189, 192–193; trends for, 164, 178, 195–196; value added by, 157–158, 160–162, 165–166, 174–176, 187–188; voluntary, 180, 197–203. *See also* Governance

Brown, M., 21, 38, 39, 116, 130, 131, 148, 171, 177–178, 197, 237, 250, 269

Brown, R., 149

Burnett, B., 120

Burns, L. R., 32, 39

C

California: group practice in, 271–272; health care plan in, 23; managed care plans in, 86

44–53, 222–223, 269–272; characteristics of successful, 232–233; chief executives of, 219–236; and community development, 280–281; conclusion on, 67; establishing purpose and mission of, 173–174; ethical dilemmas for, 138, 143–144; and ethical relationships with physicians, 92–103; financing, 233, 235, 271, 273; future for, 56–60; and global budgeting, 53–55; governance of, 153–215; institutional goals of, 161; issues for, 221–225; and joint ventures, 201–202, 239; and managed care, 32–34; and Medicare, 71–73; national chains of, 25, 33–34, 81–82; nonprofit, 78–80; operating results for, 181–182; ownership of, 32–33, 120–121; principles for, 58, 60; and reasonable costs, 50; regulation and market factors for, 33, 46–50; responsibilities of, 4; and risk shifting, 16; role of, 184–186; statistics on, 44–45; trends for, 36–37, 69, 78–84; trust in, 40–67; utilization rates for, 82–84, 87. *See also* Providers

Human resources, graduate programs in, 265

Humana: and managed care, 33; ownership of, 198

I

Ideas, power of, 22, 27

Illness intensity, and capitation, 16

Independent practice associations (IPAs), in economic era, 5

Information systems, graduate programs in, 264–265

InPhyNet, 34–35

Insurers: accountability for, 146; and capitation, 109; and catastrophic coverage, 62, 64; change for, 270, 274, 278; and community rating

basis, 54–55; ethical dilemmas for, 138–139; and health promotion, 253; and managed care, 30–31, 33; and reasonable costs, 51; trends for, 35–36, 118, 124, 134, 136

Integrated health care system (IHCS): aspects of governance for, 204–215; background on, 204–205; and community responsibility, 209; conclusions on, 215; graduate programs for, 258–266; and individual autonomy, 210–211; and local autonomy, 209–210; and managed care, 207–208; management role in, 208–209, 211–215; profit status of, 205–207; trend for, 178, 193

Integration: horizontal and vertical, 28; regional, 22; vertical, and physicians, 238. *See also* Affiliations

Interstudy, 74, 75n, 76n, 91

Investor-owned institutions, regional integration of, 22

J

Johnson, E. A., 40, 92, 131, 137, 258

Johnson, R. L., 3, 40, 68, 107, 130, 131, 155, 170, 172–179, 180, 204, 219, 238, 249, 270

Johnson administration, 23

Johnson & Johnson (J&J), and merged organizations, 25

Joint ventures: and ethics, 94, 96, 97, 100; hospitals in, 201–202, 239

K

Kaiser, H., 280

Kaiser Foundation Plan, and costs, 121

Kaiser-Permanente: and community development, 280–281; culture of, 17, 210; and institutional goals, 161, 199; staff model of, 31